Secrets of Pain

The Hidden Meaning of Symptoms

Robert L. Janda, MA, DC

For information contact:
Dr. Robert L. Janda, MA, DC
www.NaturalCureDoctor.com
2025 Newport Blvd. Suite 110, Costa Mesa, CA 92627
Tel: 714-323-4496

ISBN-13: 978-1466286887

DEDICATION

This book is dedicated to George Goodheart, DC for his amazing discoveries in Applied Kinesiology.

Contents

Robert L. Janda, MA, DC

Chapter-1

Background Concepts

Perspectives on Pain

Not everything that is going wrong in the body hurts. Some individuals discover they have Cancer with little warning. Sometimes individuals will have their bodies give out for no apparent reason. For example, reaching for something and collapsing as the low back gives out. When these cases are investigated, we will always find dysfunctions that preceded the appearance of the manifest problems. Therefore, only emphasizing disease and even pain misses the multitude of dysfunctions that were present before the disease emerged. Usually we summarize health problems under a diagnosis, like Sciatica or Parkinson's.

It is as though the individual "got Sciatica" or "got Parkinson's Disease," when in fact, the disease is a synthesis of failed functions. This synthesis of failed functions is a new organization of the body representing an attempt to function within new limitations, much like a limp is an attempt to walk while avoiding pain. The natural healer works backward trying to uncover and revive these underlying functions to reestablish health.

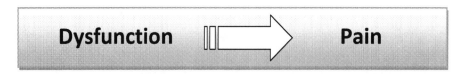

Dysfunction ⟹ **Pain**

If we resolve the dysfunctions in the mental, physiological and structural areas, pain and disease often disappear on their own. Therefore, it is wise to regard the road from dysfunction to pain and disease as a continuum. This concept is old in Natural Medicine, yet it is evolving in the emerging field of Functional Medicine, which uses the tools of science to understand the dysfunctions that lead to health problems. This approach will clearly play an expanding role as time moves on. In the case histories to follow, we will make some effort to show the dysfunctions that are underlying the symptoms.

Underlying Reflexes Related to Pain

I am a Chiropractor and people usually come to me because they are experiencing pain somewhere in the body. They usually explain their problem by indicating that they hurt themselves by "twisting something" or "pulling something," the assumption being that the pain is some sort of sprain or strain. While these kinds of injuries do often occur, it is rarely the full story. We can make a distinction between primary dysfunction of a joint due to trauma or a repetitive strain to the joint itself, and secondary dysfunction of a joint whose cause is located somewhere else in the body. As far as joints are concerned, the traumatic injuries are often the most serious, usually leading to degeneration if left untreated. However, they are not the most common. Most painful areas in the body are hurting due to referred pain, that is, pain referred from another area that is having problems, and which may or may not in itself hurt. The inside of the body and the outside are mysteriously linked together in a secret partnership.

Why would the body do this? Why doesn't it just hurt where the problem is? This is an important question because its answer has implications for developing a strategy to correct the cause of the pain. We will attempt to answer this by exploring some concepts from Chinese Medicine. In acupuncture theory, there are two classifications of acupuncture points that we will explore here.

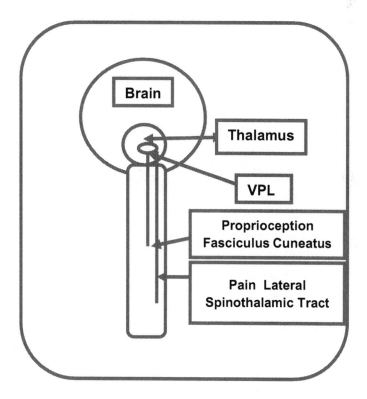

One group is called Association Points, and the other group is called Alarm Points. Association Points are points on the Bladder

Meridian and are located on the back in two rows right along the spine. Alarm Points, on the other hand, are located on the front of the body. Both sets of points reflect disturbances in organ systems within the body. In Western Medicine, both of these points are thought of as Viscera-Somatic Reflexes, meaning reflexes that connect the internal organs to the Musculoskeletal System. In Western Medicine, this concept is a general one and is noted for such things as pain shooting down the arm from a heart attack, or shoulder pain from a Gallbladder Dysfunction. In Chinese Medicine, this concept is more extensively refined with both front and back specific points reflecting internal dysfunction. But why have both front and back points reflecting internal dysfunction? Why not just have one? Traditionally, the Association Points on the back are thought to reflect more chronic conditions, and the Alarm Points on the front are thought to reflect acute conditions. I will illustrate that they have different functions. Alarm Points and Association Points are not really doing the same thing. That is why there are two sets of points on the body.

Association Points

Let's start with the Association Points on the back. Say your liver hurts and the Association Point connected with the liver, Bladder 18 at the level of the 9th Thoracic Vertebra, becomes sore. Why would the body make that point sore? It is known that soreness of an Association Point is connected with a Subluxation of the vertebrae at that same level. A Subluxation is a Chiropractic concept and is defined as a mal-positioned vertebra that is causing nerve interference. We know that when a joint is out of place, out of the neutral position, it generates increasing amounts of Proprioceptive information telling the body what it is doing. Now there is an interesting relationship between Proprioception and pain. It's been noted that pain and Proprioception each travel up different pathways to the brain. But in the brain, specifically in a place called the VPL (Ventral Posterio-Lateral Nucleus of the Thalamus), both types of information meet. This means there is a competition at receptor sites for these two types of information to be received at the same location simultaneously. Why? Well, if there is competition between pain and Proprioception, then you cannot feel pain and feel Proprioception at the same time for the same area of the body. The stronger the Proprioceptive input, the less the pain. Why would that be?

Imagine you are a deer who is being attacked by a lion. As long as you are moving and Proprioceptive information is being generated, you suppress pain. This action keeps pain from distracting your efforts to escape, leaving your brain clear to deal with the dangerous situation. When the famous explorer, Dr. Livingston was attacked by a lion in Africa, he said it did not hurt at all.

Here's another example. Suppose I see you resting comfortably in a chair and I tiptoe over without you knowing, and hit you suddenly. You would be jolted and sit up in shock, angry and disturbed, and it might take hours for you to calm down.

Now imagine you are in that same chair and I walk up and tell you I am going to hit you. You grit your teeth and tighten your body. Now when I hit you it has little effect.

The Proprioception from clenching your muscles suppressed the shock of the blow. In a few minutes you are back to normal. So when we see a functional Subluxation in the spine we know the body is trying to suppress pain for the sake of mental clarity.

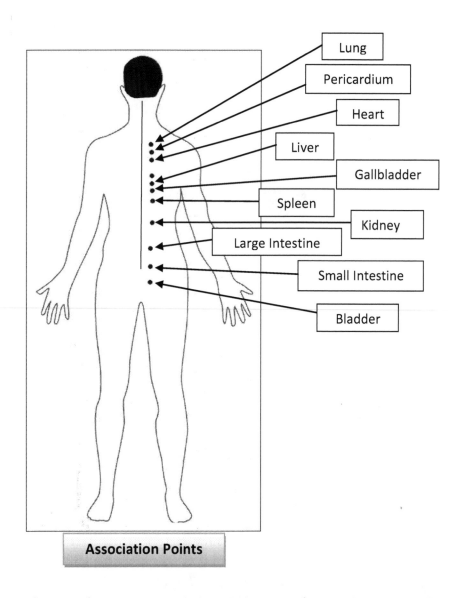

Association Points

That is the way Association Points work as Viscerosomatic Reflexes. If these reflexes did not exist you would be subject to jolting pain shocks from inside your body. The reason why Traditional Acupuncture regards these as points reflecting chronic conditions is that in acute conditions the Proprioceptive information is usually produced by motion. As the condition becomes more chronic the Proprioception is generated by Subluxation, thus activating the Association Points. So if functional Subluxations are such a gift for clearing our mind why are Chiropractors constantly trying to get rid of them? That is another story and will be explained later.

Alarm Points

Now let's look at the Alarm Points on the front of the body. These occur within the soft tissues, between ribs or on the abdomen, and do not involve joints, this is a critical difference. There is a Proprioceptive function involved with these points also, but most are imbedded in the soft tissue on the front of the body and serve a different function. Unlike the Association Points which are clustered along the spinal column, the Alarm Points are usually situated right over the organ they refer to. The liver point is located over the liver, the heart point over the heart, etc. Alarm Points will always inhibit the muscles that run through them, as well as the muscle chains that run through them. This is easy to demonstrate with Muscle Testing. One of the main characteristics of Alarm Points is that they are painful, and they hurt even more when the muscle and Fascial tissues in which they are imbedded are stretched. Therefore, a person will avoid stretching an active Alarm Point by leaning towards it if it becomes very sore. We see this when someone is running and gets a "stitch" in the side. This is an organ inflammation that results in an Alarm Point being flared up. The person will put his hand over the Alarm Point and lean towards it. What advantage does this have? When you lean towards an Alarm Point you relax the Fascia around the organ associated with it. This takes pressure off the organ, increases circulation and provides a better chance of healing. So Alarm Points function to direct posture and inhibit compression of the involved organ.

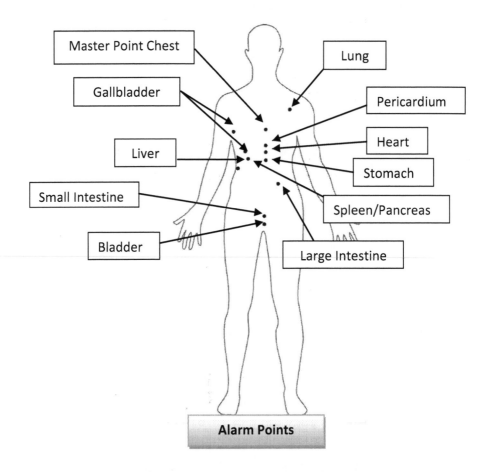

Alarm Points

They inhibit the muscles that cross an inflamed organ. By inhibiting these muscles, the Alarm Points prevent compression of the organ that occurs when the muscles contract. That makes sense, but why don't the organs themselves hurt to serve the same function? I propose that the Alarm Points serve the function of driving the cues for pain adaptation centripetally, away from the core to make the direction for postural adjustment more obvious to the nervous system.

In summary, both Association Points and Alarm Points hurt, but serve different functions. Association Points calm the mind in the face of pain, and Alarm Points help protect the inflamed organ from muscular compression. Both have influence on posture, but Alarm Points more so.

Association Points usually involve joint inflammation from joint mal-position, and inflamed joints do not like compression. In severe cases, the posturing will be to lean away from the inflamed joint. In less severe cases, the Malposition of the joint is usually a fixation of the vertebrae in a rotated position at that level. Although this does result in a minor postural distortion, the spine usually compensates for this by rotating another vertebrae farther up the spine in the opposite direction. This is called a "Lovett Brother Relationship" in Applied Kinesiology. This will correct the postural distortion.

Alarm Points, on the other hand, are imbedded in soft tissue and are not related to joints. Because inflamed tissue does not like to be stretched, an individual will tend to lean towards the pain to relieve it. This additionally promotes healing of the affected organ by protecting it against compression. This relieves Fascial stress on the organ, which helps with circulation and healing.

These two patterns of pain avoidance will have different ramifications for the way symptoms are displayed as we focus on specific areas of pain. In addition, both types of points will affect pain awareness. Association Points will sedate nerve pain signals to the brain by competitive inhibition of Proprioception and pain, and Alarm Points function by changing posture to reduce pain output from an inflamed organ.

Trigger Points and Ah Shi Points

Both Ah Shi and Trigger Points refer to painful areas that appear at various places on the surface of the body as an expression of physiological and postural abnormalities. Ah Shi Points are not distinguished from Trigger Points in Chinese Medicine, although they appear to have a different function. Trigger Points are painful nodules imbedded in muscle tissue that support muscle contraction without conscious awareness, thus allowing for "effortless chronic contraction."

Causes of Pain – Unrecognized Infection

This book is not designed to be a reference textbook that systematically covers different possibilities for the various problems illustrated here, but rather to present the most common causes of manifest pain as I have encountered them in my practice. Not infrequently, a sizable number of these patients have seen other doctors, Medical and Chiropractic, and have not responded to care. This is largely because the vast majority of doctors view their patients through a filter of ideas they have learned. Unless these ideas are reexamined if and when they fail, the patient will move from doctor to doctor with little or no result. The ideas presented here have proven to be useful in alleviating the ailments experienced by the majority of patients that I see. But apparently many doctors do not utilize them or these patients would have responded to their care and subsequently would not have needed to inquire about my Chiropractic services for the same condition.

There are multiple causes for pain manifestation including disruption of the physical structure of the body, misuse of the body, toxins, circulation problems, infection and others. Infection has always been present as a source of pain, but has recently become so common that it has now become my patients' top priority. Microbes are on the rise all over the world and will probably continue to ascend until we have a great plague and humans once again become serious about controlling them. Right now, economic interests are dominant and infections travel freely around the globe. Microbes are transported on food, tourists, insect vectors, animals and other means. So they increasingly show up everywhere in our lives and cause an excess of maladies. Most of these infections are subclinical; meaning that, aside from seemingly unrelated symptoms, such as aches and Viscerosomatic Reflexes, there is little sign of infection. The truth is that the technology for finding subclinical infections is still not very evolved. Such a major disease as Rheumatoid Arthritis may well be due to infection, as I believe it is, yet the bulk of the Medical field believes it is due to autoimmune causes and treats the problem by attempting to suppress the immune system. Yet, as far as I am aware, the most effective approach has been that of Thomas Mc Pearson Brown, M.D. who has treated over 10,000 cases successfully using Tetracycline for infection. That such a prominent disease could be subject to this debate illustrates the difficulty in identifying infection. As in this case, a doctor must often make a decision how to proceed without definitive information. Alternative techniques such as Applied Kinesiology or Muscle Testing and new forms of computerized electrical analysis of the body, such as Voll Testing or LSA (Limbic Stress Assessment) Tests, offer dramatic new ways of exposing infection. These technologies evaluate electrical frequency signals from the body to screen for disturbances. Many individuals believe simple lab testing will do the job. In my experience, this has not been the case.

To give some idea of the problem, there are perhaps 2,400 types of Trematodes, which are microscopic worms. The body will sense their presence and produce chemicals to fight them called antibodies. Although there are thousands of types of Trematodes, there are only half a dozen antibody tests. A positive Antibody Test is useful because it confirms the body is fighting, or has fought, a Trematode infection, but what does a negative test mean? It might indicate that there isn't any infection, but it also might mean that infection is present but goes undetected because we have no antibody test for it. Stool tests are also very inaccurate as the infection may be predominately in the organs of the body. Frequently, antibody tests and stool tests do not agree with each other. Presently, a doctor must be a detective to find hidden infections, and this problem will continue until the technology improves.

Viscero-Somatic Reflexes

From what I have written above, it should be clear that disturbances within the body affect the Musculo-Skeletal System. These effects include what has already been discussed; such phenomena as Alarm Points, Association Points, Subluxations and Ah Shi or Trigger Points. These can all be viewed as examples of Viscera-Somatic Reflexes. Aside from the above examples, another common manifestation of a Viscero-Somatic Reflex is muscle spasm. This is readily recognized whenever there is inflammation, and it is not limited to organ inflammation. Any joint or muscle that is inflamed will often cause muscle spasm and I hope to illustrate this in the case histories to follow. In this context, muscle spasm is a guarding reflex to protect the injured area from becoming worse. However, the muscle spasm is rigid and blocks motion. Lack of motion prevents proper circulation of blood and Lymph and over time further irritates inflammation. Thus it is a somewhat self defeating strategy. This is due to a conflict between the short term benefits and the long term consequences of constricting muscle spasm.

We also see changes in blood flow, Vasodilation and Vaso-Constriction. These reflexes are also triggered by toxins, inflammation, infection and other factors. These reflexes can lead to pain because the effects of blood flow are essential for proper body function and to establish homeostasis.

We can regard Viscerosomatic Reflexes as an expression of a wide variety of underlying disturbances that can be toxic, infectious, inflammatory, stress induced or due to deficiencies of needed nutrients. Obviously, the deepest therapeutic response to these expressions is to identify the nature of the underlying disturbance and correct it. However, another therapeutic approach that is often employed is to help the body adapt to these stresses in the hope that it would be able to fix itself. Therapies such as Acupuncture, Massage and Chiropractic Manipulation are of this nature. These respectively influence energetics, blood and Lymph flow, and nerve interference. There is no doubt that they provide a genuine benefit. It is often advantageous to use more than one of these approaches, as they most probably are synergistic in their effects. At the moment, the choice of therapies is an art form requiring considerable clinical experience, as we presently have no available research to discriminate what pattern of therapies would be most beneficial.

Chapter - 2

Natural Healing

In general, Natural Healing is the most philosophically coherent and practical method of responding to the maladies of life, for both animals and people. This is because the tools it uses for healing are either natural for the body, such as food, or have co-evolved with the chemical systems in the body, such as herbs. The result of using these types of medicines is that there are few side effects to the treatment. Natural Healing also attempts to understand the matrix of health problems, such as diet and psychological stress, and works to correct the problem at its source.

Natural Healing is healing that is based on promoting the innate ability of the body to heal itself by utilizing natural sources such as food, manual manipulation and herbs. Allopathic Medicine is modern medicine based on the use of artificial drugs and disease attacking strategies such as surgery or radiation. There is no absolute line to draw between Natural Healing and Allopathic Medicine, but there is a very significant difference in emphasis.

Allopathic Medicine tends to identify problems in terms of discrete diagnosis and prescribe a treatment for the disease.

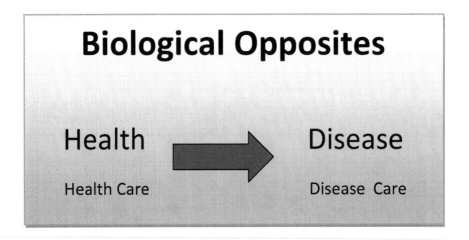

Natural Healing searches for underlying dysfunctions which cumulatively lead to pathology. The treatment is directed at the underlying dysfunctions rather than at the disease. As an example, cardiovascular disease is usually treated by Allopathic Medicine by targeting Cholesterol and fats in the blood and prescribing drugs to reduce them, such as Statins. Natural Healing focuses on the reasons for high blood fats, including high saturated and trans fats, by looking at the diet as a cause. And it focuses on causes of inflammation such as infection, lack of good fats, acidic diet and toxins. It may also seek to correct hormonal deficiencies. Cholesterol is a precursor to steroid hormones and the body may be increasing Cholesterol to make more hormones. Natural Healing may also explore stress and exercise as factors in plaque formation. It may evaluate antioxidant status, such as using Vitamin C to help prevent Cholesterol from being oxidized, and so on. None of these produce any side effects and only strengthen the body. The famous US Civil Rights Lawyer, Jonathan Emord, has commented that most supplements are less toxic than food. Allopathic treatments have their most relevance in emergency medicine, or at the limits of our understanding of Natural Healing. The use of Statin drugs in Allopathic Medicine, on the other hand, can cause dizziness, nausea, bloating, diarrhea, headaches, muscle soreness and a loss of Co-Enzyme Q-10. There are benefits to these drugs, but we need to ask if these substances are really healthy to take, especially when there are other healthy alternatives available.

Two Types of Care

We might consider Health and Sickness to be on a continuum with no sharp boundary between them. The United States spends more per capita than any country in the world on health care, yet is ranked 37th in health status. This fact alone should give us pause regarding our attitude towards healing. This is largely due to almost exclusive funding of the disease model of doctoring and political enforcement of these views. If we can assume American doctors do not have a lower IQ than those in the rest of the world, then it must be due to the politics of our system. The primary intention of Natural Medicine is to build health. The primary intention of Allopathic Medicine is to fight disease. The concepts and knowledge base for each are different, although they overlap, especially in areas of basic science. Most of the efforts of Natural Medicine are to facilitate and amplify the natural healing mechanisms within the body.

It is often assumed that medicine will eventually understand everything and all illness will be cured. I believe this is a fundamental error in thinking. While it is true that the absolute amount of knowledge increases each year and has filled libraries, it appears the ratio of knowledge to ignorance never changes. I don't believe we are any better off than the cave men in this regard. Each new bit of knowledge brings forth new questions, equations, and new consequences that need further investigation. This will never end. As the Yin/Yang symbol indicates reality is always made half of light and half of dark. Therefore, any approach to healing should involve some way of relating to the unknown and the uncertain. This should start with a respect for natural process in the body which already expresses a long history of adaptation to the challenges of life and the ever present uncertainty in which we exist.

Muscle Testing

Some discussion of Applied Kinesiology Muscle Testing is in order here, since much reference will be made to it in this writing. I would like to say first, that Muscle Testing is a new discipline and has only recently started to be investigated scientifically. It has primarily been developed through clinical observation. Muscle Testing has many critics, some who have a venomous attitude, regarding it as unproven nonsense without any foundation in reality, promoted by gullible quacks lost in fantasy. This is not true. However, like any new area of investigation the clinical models vastly outstrip the science behind it. Therefore, we should not confuse scientific validation with truth. Many fields have been developed to a high degree and later investigated scientifically. Note the ideas in Psychoanalysis later translated into learning theory by Dollard and Miller. Note the nutritional Cancer treatment developed by Max Gerson, M.D. The medical field took away his medical license for quackery, which was later reinstated by the US Senate after viewing the evidence he presented in his book, "A Cancer Therapy: Results of Fifty Cases and the Cure of Advanced Cancer". Note also the fields of Herbology, Acupuncture and

Chiropractic. Both Acupuncture and Chiropractic have been regarded skeptically by the medical profession for a century. Only when former President Nixon returned from China with videos of individuals undergoing major surgery with only Acupuncture anesthesia did we realize our views were highly opinionated and not based on fact. Likewise, studies on Chiropractic done by the British, Canadian and US Governments have proven the value of manipulation therapy. While the point is well taken that someone making claims has the burden of proof on them, it is also reasonable to expect the scientific evolution of these techniques to take some time. In the meanwhile, the effectiveness of clinical practice should provide a basis for their appreciation. As clinicians we do not primarily function as scientists. Science is a particular game for building models of reality based on testable hypotheses. When it comes to making a decision for a particular patient, any good doctor would use what he thinks will work, whether there is science available or not. Most use of drugs is done this way. The studies of the effects of a drug on the body are based on single drugs, almost never of combinations. But almost all drugs are used in combination. This makes clinical sense to the doctor, but is not scientific. Yet, the same individuals who do this every day are critical of holistic techniques as being unscientific. Even surgery can be subject to the illusion of being scientific. A recent study on knee surgery found that some of these surgeries were no more effective than not doing the surgery at all.

It also seems to have escaped notice by its medical critics that, while they feel Muscle Testing lacks scientific validity, the same can be said about the criticisms of it. The most opinionated individuals have generated few, if any, studies invalidating the field. They just "know" through intuitive enlightenment that the field is absurd. With this kind of insight, why bother with science at all? Not all knowledge is logical and can be deduced from existing ideas. In fact, we are all trapped by the illusion of interpreting new ideas through our established concepts. Sometimes this can become worse with more education. Education does not always help you perceive completely new things that are outside your educational framework.

Some of the most interesting studies supporting the amazing potentials of Muscle Testing come, not from a Chiropractor, but from a Japanese Medical Doctor, Dr. Yoshiaki Omura. He was able to patent "Bi-Digital O-Ring Testing" with the US Patent Office, based on the evidence he presented. Unless the critics of Muscle Testing regard the US Patent Office as gullible, the evidence should be regarded with amazement. Dr. Omura had his associates, heads of Medical Schools and University Departments, design studies testing the validity of O-Ring Muscle Testing. Using this method of Muscle Testing they were able to predict the outcomes of Imaging Tests for lung Cancer, including the location of the Cancer and its type. They were able to successfully screen for stomach Cancer, later confirmed by conventional testing. They were able to diagnose pancreatic Cancer and its location within the pancreas. They were able to correctly diagnose infections with Chlamydia trachomatis, later confirmed with lab testing. They were able to correctly identify the type and location of specific neurotransmitters on prepared slides of nervous tissue. This data can be viewed at Dr. Omura's website: http://bdort.org/. The US Patent Office rejected his patent grant for years because his claims "seemed impossible" at that time. We owe our gratitude to this wonderful and visionary man.

However, Dr. Omura did not originate this conceptual use of Muscle Testing. The original concept of using Muscle Testing as a source of unusual information about the body was the brain child of Dr. George Goodheart, a Chiropractor. His insights have led to the development of the field of Applied Kinesiology within Chiropractic. The impact of his ideas has spread to related disciplines around the world. I believe Muscle Testing will eventually prove to be as valuable as X-Ray or MRI technology in clinical practice. Studies confirming its validity for Chiropractic can be found at the website for the International College of Applied Kinesiology: www.icak.com. Muscle Testing is a complex skill and anyone who uses it in his practice may spend his whole life improving his skills and exploring its ramifications.

Chapter - 3

Case Histories

Case #1 Mid-Back Pain

My secretary knocked on the door of my treatment room and informed me that a long term patient of mine had arrived in the clinic unannounced suffering from acute back pain. My secretary asked if I could please see him now!

I walked into the waiting room to find Mike standing by the front desk. I gestured him to follow me back to the treatment room and noticed he could hardly move and walked with very short shuffling steps and a very stiff body. When he arrived in the room, I asked him where it hurt. I found he would only whisper to me as he was afraid if he took a deep breath his back would go into seizure. He whispered to me that it hurt across his mid back and he had somehow thrown it out of place, the worst he had ever injured it. I asked what he had done and he told me he woke up that way and must have "slept wrong". He could hardly breathe because the pain was so severe. He had no other symptoms.

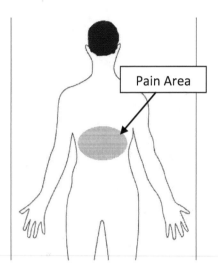

I have seen variations of this problem so many times. In fact, I was pretty sure what the problem was when I saw him standing in the waiting room. However, I proceeded to examine him using Muscle Testing. As unusual as it might at first sound, I believed he was suffering from bacterial food poisoning which had metastasized to his kidneys. Muscle Testing confirmed this; both his intestinal tract and kidneys were infected. The muscular spasm he was experiencing in his mid back was a Viscera-Somatic reflex from his kidneys producing "Guarding Reflexes."

Guarding Reflexes are muscle spasms produced by the body in an attempt to immobilize an injured area to protect it from further injury. The poison from the bacteria had also inflamed his joints, nerves and muscles; much like the flu makes your body stiff. There was no point in attempting spinal manipulation when he was in that condition, so I carefully sat him in a chair and fed him a large dose of Probiotics, a serving of about 100 billion. These are living bacteria that belong in the intestinal tract and are territorial. A dose of this size will quickly overwhelm the pathogenic bacteria and, in a short time, restore normal intestinal flora. This restoration, in fact, happened. In about 30 minutes, his symptoms became so minimal he was able to move with little discomfort. Usually cases like this take a few hours to resolve, but I was happy to see him respond so quickly, and we soon said good-by.

While this is a severe case, it is also typical. In my practice perhaps 80% or more of people with mid back pain have infected kidneys and it is usually bacterial. The usual symptoms are just a feeling of stiffness in the mid back without manifest pain. Most kidney infections are secondary to intestinal infection, and this is commonly true of other infected organs as well. Usually when the intestinal infection is corrected the metastatic infection to the organ will die out on its own.

Case #2 Knee Pain

Sarah explained to me that her right knee pain was getting so bad that she had trouble getting up and down the stairs in her house. This had been going on for several weeks. She did not remember specifically injuring her knee, it just started hurting and had been gradually getting worse. She went to her Medical Doctor who told her she had strained her knee and prescribed pain killers to use if she needed them. When I examined the knee I didn't find any specific problem with the knee itself. It moved easily and palpation did not reveal inflammation in the soft tissue surrounding it.

One clue was that it hurt mainly when she ascended or descended stairs. This suggested muscular involvement. When I started testing the muscles surrounding the knee, I found the Rectus Femoris weak. This is a muscle that attaches both at the knee cap and at the hip, crossing two joints.

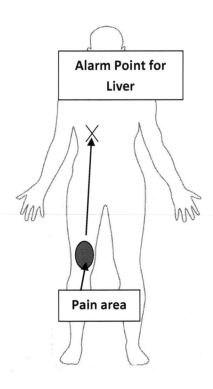

Why would this muscle be weak? I know that there are supportive and stabilizing muscles for the Rectus Femoris in both the stomach area and the chest, so I started looking for organs that may be inflamed and causing reflex weakening of this muscle. Sure enough, Muscle Testing revealed the liver was inflamed. In fact, when the patient held her hand over this organ, the Rectus Femoris became instantly strong. This told me that the liver was inflamed and it was directly connected to the weakening of this muscle. But why was the liver inflamed?

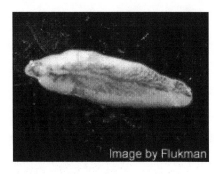

Image by Flukman

There are a number of possibilities causing liver inflammation, but the most common are fatty foods causing liver congestion, or infection. The patient told me she had not been eating fatty foods, so I decided this was not likely to be a productive line of investigation. Also, the patient had not been drinking alcohol which might irritate the liver. I decided next to test for infection. After Muscle Testing for a number of possibilities the testing suggested this individual had a low grade infection of liver flukes or Trematodes. These are small microscopic parasitic worms that look like little leaves, flat and pointed at both ends, and have become quite common in the United States in the past few years. I know from experience that running a stool test to confirm this will take weeks and will likely be negative since the infection is minor and imbedded in the liver, not the intestine. Usually, stool tests will only show positive for flukes if the infection is significant and it involves the intestine. The other major form of testing that may be useful is Antibody Testing. If the body has a particular type of infection, a class of white cells called Lymphocytes will start manufacturing chemicals called antibodies to attack the flukes.

Even if these organisms cannot be directly located and seen, antibody tests may indicate the body is or has been fighting this organism. However, this kind of testing also takes weeks. Another problem is that there are about 2,400 types of Trematodes and only a handful of antibody tests, making the likelihood high of a negative result. Since the infection was subclinical I decided to treat her with herbs that would help the body eliminate this parasite. I sent the patient home with some Artemisia, an herb helpful for various types of worms, and had her come back in four days. When she returned four days later her knee pain was gone and, in fact, had disappeared two days earlier.   The Rectus Femoris now tested strong, confirming what I had thought; the knee hurt because the liver was inflamed.

These types of problems are quite common. It may involve the liver, or it may involve any other organ along the line of support for muscles associated with the knee, such as the lungs or heart. Subclinical bacterial food poisoning is the most common cause of spontaneous knee pain, in my experience. There are also numerous other possibilities which are beyond the scope of this essay to describe. These types of cases usually do not respond to physical therapy. The therapists are very disadvantaged treating this as a knee strain instead of as a reflex inhibition of supporting muscles of the knee. As a general rule, if a muscle is inhibited reflexively and engaged in activity, the origins and insertions of the muscle are likely to become sore. This is what is interpreted as knee pain in this case.

I have found this kind of thinking very useful for understanding joint problems throughout the body. These kinds of symptoms can mimic those from repetitive strain injuries or even trauma. It can be confusing if one joint is injured from trauma and the next from reflexive problems unrelated to the problem. Sometimes the same joint has more than one source for its symptoms.

Case #3 Shoulder Pain

This was a strange case of a Mexican woman in her early 30s who came in complaining of left shoulder pain. Her shoulder had started hurting several weeks before and had gotten progressively worse. She reported that she thought she hurt it house cleaning as the soreness started after a long day of work. She seemed to be able to move the shoulder in all directions, but stiffly and painfully. She pointed to her shoulder in the vicinity of the rotator cuff when I asked her to describe where the pain was worst.

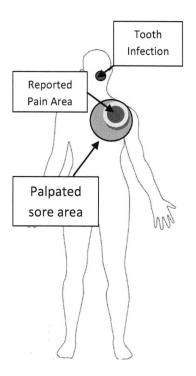

However, none of the rotator cuff muscles tested weak. The rotator cuff area did elicit pain with palpation, but I soon discovered the rest of the shoulder hurt also. I started applying pressure to delineate the total area of pain and found it extended down her upper arm and also into her chest and axilla. Because the chest area was so sore I became concerned she had a lung tumor or infection. She reported she had no signs of infection, so I sent her for a chest x-ray. She returned two days later, but the x-ray was negative. At this point, I started checking her with Muscle Testing for infection. To my surprise she tested positive for bacterial infection over the wide area of her shoulder and muscles of her chest. I asked if she felt sick, had run a fever, of if the shoulder had become hot. She insisted she was fine. I started checking the rest of her body for infection and everything checked negative. I was perplexed. Almost never does an infection show up in a major joint without also showing up in other areas of the body, particularly the intestinal tract. Her intestines were fine, so were her kidneys, bladder, liver and pancreas. I rechecked her shoulder and chest and the same infection was present as noted. I began questioning her again, going over the same material, but this time her husband had come in to watch. They started speaking in Spanish, and in a moment he asked me if a root canal counted. Of course it did! I had forgotten to check her teeth using Kinesiology. She had a low grade root canal infection that had spread to her shoulder. The infection was not bad enough to cause the usual signs of infection in her mouth cavity, but infection was present nevertheless. I sent her to her dentist and her shoulder pain went away within two days after receiving treatment from him. This is a good illustration of how something that seemed like a sprain or strain was really something else.

Case #4 Low Back Pain

A young woman in her early 20s drove a hundred miles to see me from Palm Springs. She was suffering from low back pain and she felt she had exhausted the medical, acupuncture and

Chiropractic resources in her area. Nobody could figure out why her back hurt. She had been thoroughly examined, including X-Rays and an MRI, but all were negative. She came such a long way because I had treated her brother successfully for a shoulder pain that also had not been resolved by resources where they lived.

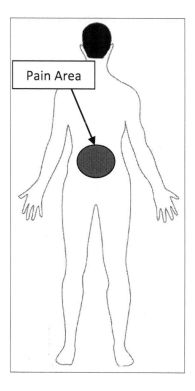

This pain in her back had been going on for a few months and had slowly been getting worse. It was interfering with sleep and college, and her grades were starting to suffer (she was a straight A student). Indeed, her low back was in spasm and the vertebrae and sacroiliac joints in her pelvis were sore to pressure. Orthopedic tests indicated a general stiffness, but no focal acute pain. Nearly all the muscles in her legs were weak when tested. Further testing revealed they were all strengthened when she placed her hand over her abdomen.

This is a phenomenon called Therapy Localization in the Chiropractic field of Applied Kinesiology. What this means is that touching a disturbed area of the body will weaken any strong muscle in the body, as well as strengthen a weak one that is involved with the problem. It does not tell you what the problem is, only where. I then set out to discover what was wrong with her abdomen. Muscle Testing revealed she was suffering from a parasite infection. I did not have the AK Test Kits available to determine more specifically what the infection was, only that it was a Protozoa infection. I sent her for a Comprehensive Stool Test and two weeks later the result came back that she was severely infected by a Protozoa called Dientamoeba Fragilis, a small flagellated microbe similar to Giardia. I referred her back to her Medical Doctor for treatment, but they were not familiar with treating this parasite. I referred her to another Medical Doctor I know who is a specialist in infectious disease. Her treatment took several months and got worse before she recovered. In the process she was forced to drop out of college. (She has since graduated).

This was another case that appeared to be a sprain or strain or a disc problem, but was, in fact, another infection. I have seen this many times.

Case #5 Abdominal Pain with Low Back Pain

This is a particularly strange case because of the length of time the symptoms had been going on. This was a 70-year-old woman who had been suffering from abdominal pain and low back pain for 30 years! She had been treated by doctors for that condition during the entire 30 year period, including many bouts of antibiotic treatments. Nothing had worked, except for short term partial relief. As low back pains are often associated with abdominal stress,

I assumed this was likely the root of both her problems. This was particularly true given her long medical history.

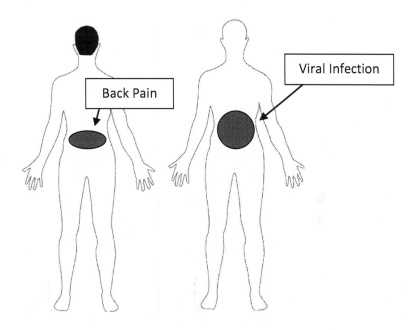

Her abdomen tested positive with Muscle Testing for Viral Infection. There was no point in further evaluation until this issue was resolved, so I gave her a supplement with Gamma Globulins which are effective against abdominal viruses.

The entire exam and treatment recommendation took about two minutes. She commented, half joking, that I was certainly charging her for my time, although I only charged her my minimum fee. She left, but two days later I got a message from her friend that her pain had gone away for the first time ever.

This case illustrates the Viscera-Somatic Reflex to the back muscles from the abdomen. It also shows that simple lab testing such as stool tests and blood tests do not always reveal low grade infections, even ones that are long standing. It also shows how useful Muscle Testing can be in these cases.

Case #6 Achilles Tendonitis

Jane was a hiker and complained that she developed pain in her Achilles Tendon after a couple of miles of hiking. If she rested it for a few days the pain went away, but would return as soon as she started hiking again. She wanted to know what was wrong.

In thinking about these kinds of problems it is helpful to know about a common clinical observation; that reflexive interference with a muscle will often lead to pain at the origin or insertion of that muscle. The Achilles Tendon forms the insertion for both the Gastrocnemius and the Soleus muscles in the calf. Therefore, we first wondered if there is anything interfering with these muscles. How would we test this? Using AK Muscle Testing this is easy to do. We know that muscles function in chains, as we already discussed, so we would expect the hamstrings to be part of the Soleus/Gastrocnemius pattern. So we turn the patient face down and test the hamstrings, which are strong. We then had Jane dorsiflex her foot while testing the hamstring (this stretches the Achilles Tendon). When we do this we find it weakens the hamstring. So we know that this muscle chain does not function well together.

Next, we look for the source of the reflex interference. To make the story short we know that the kidneys are in the line of muscle support for the hamstring muscles. Muscle Testing indicates the kidney is disturbed with an infection. When we touch the area over the kidney, the hamstring tests strong (even with the foot dorsiflexed).

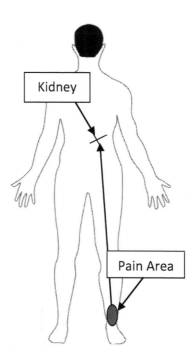

Touching an area of the body puts energy into that area of the body and can change the reflex pattern. When we take our hand off the kidney, the hamstring again becomes weak. This tells us that the kidney is the source of the reflex interference to the Achilles Tendon.

Clinical experience tells us that the kidneys rarely are a primary source of infection. Most of the time kidney infections come from the intestinal tract, although there are other possibilities. So we turned Jane over and screened her intestines for infection. Just as we suspected, Muscle Testing indicated there was an infection. Now we know that the treatment for her Achilles Tendonitis is to give her several large doses of Acidophilus, the good bacteria, to get rid of the intestinal infection. Most of the time when the primary infection is eradicated (in the intestine), the secondary one (in the kidney) will disappear all on its own. There is usually a lag time of a few hours to a day or two for this to occur. We gave Jane her Acidophilus and within a day her tendonitis faded away, even during her hikes. This symptom has happened to Jane several times, so now when she develops her tendonitis she just comes in and asks for Acidophilus.

Case #7 Costo-Sternal Pain

John did not complain of rib pain. He came in for treatment for his neck. I noticed that the rib attachments to his sternum were acutely sore while working on his neck. I often rub reflex points in the chest to stimulate muscle relaxation in the neck. In his case these joints were so sore that he jumped when I put pressure on them. Soreness in these joints is more common than we might suppose. Most people do not realize these joints are inflamed unless someone puts pressure on them. Yet, they can be amazingly sore. Why would these joints become so sore?

In Chinese Medicine these points on either side of the sternum are on the Kidney Meridian. Does this offer us clues to their soreness? These joints are cartilaginous, and are different from the rib joints in the back which are regular Articular joints. The cartilage is one key to their soreness.

To understand how these joints are related to the kidneys we need to know how the Chinese thought about the Kidneys. They divide the functions of the Kidney into Kidney Yang and Kidney Yin. Kidney Yang is the active fiery aspect of the Kidney and in modern medicinal terms this refers to the Adrenal Glands, the small glands that sit on top of the Kidneys. So in Chinese Medicine the Kidneys do not just refer to the Kidney organs, but groups both the Kidneys and the Adrenal Glands under the 'Kidney' energy system.

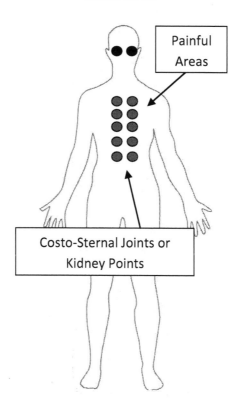

These small glands produce hormones, in particular Cortisol, Testosterone and Adrenaline, all of which have some role in stimulating metabolism. Kidney Yin refers to the fluid processing and detoxifying functions. But for our purposes here, the Adrenals are the main glands that respond to stress, producing Cortisol.

Why should stress and Cortisol affect these kidney points and make them sore? For one, during stress, the Adrenals use large amounts of Vitamin C, and the Cortisol pulls Calcium out of bones and cartilage. The Vitamin C helps build connective tissue in bones and cartilage, so in general, stress weakens cartilage and bones by preventing their repair. Poor repair of bones shows up first in these joints because the cartilage here bends slightly as the ribs move up and down with each breath. This micro-bending of the cartilage causes "use damage", much like metal fatigue (when metal is bent repeatedly it will break). Because of this, the cartilage needs constant repair. In a sense, pain in these joints is an early form of Scurvy.

However, when I used Muscle Testing to evaluate the Adrenals in this patient, I found they were not weak. While this did not indicate they were not under stress, it did suggest the stress had not been of long duration or they would have shown signs of exhaustion, and it takes a while to weaken cartilage and produce cartilage inflammation. So, why were these joints sore? We next considered the lungs. Because the lungs have so much surface area they are very prone to free radical damage from pollutants in the air, or from infection.

I have read that monkeys put in cages under a freeway overpass show lung damage within an hour from smog. Free radical exposure from the air will exhaust the lungs reserves of Beta-Carotene, Vitamin A, Vitamin C and a very important lung antioxidant called Glutathione. When we tested this patient's lungs with Applied Kinesiology evaluation they did indeed show weakness and a need for nearly all antioxidants.

This indicates something, possibly air pollution, is using up John's antioxidants including the Vitamin C that is needed to repair his Costo-Sternal joints. I recommended he take a number of antioxidants, but I also included L-Cystine. As I mentioned, this is the primary limiting ingredient in forming Glutathione, which is so important for protecting the lungs. Within three or four weeks the soreness faded from the cartilage in his chest.

Case #8 Carpal Tunnel Pain

A young woman named Lin came to me with bilateral wrist pain. She had been diagnosed with Carpal Tunnel by two Orthopedists and surgery had been recommended by both. She did not want surgery. A friend told her about our office and she came in for an "alternative" opinion. Lin did exhibit weakness in the grip of both hands and soreness was produced while tapping the Carpal Tunnel, indicating the nerve was irritated at that location. It was difficult to hold a pencil or use a computer mouse. This was a classical case of Carpal Tunnel.

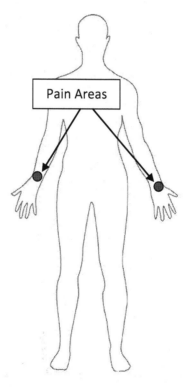

Carpal Tunnel needs some explanation as there is a large discrepancy between the medical model of this problem and what science and clinical evidence now knows to be the cause of this painful condition. The well established medical model envisions the median nerve being entrapped under the transverse ligament of the wrist causing inflammation of the nerve along with weakness of the enervated muscles.

This makes logical sense, that the carpal tunnel collapses and the median nerve is entrapped under the transverse ligament causing pain and tingling. Insurance companies have accepted this explanation and routinely pay the bills for surgery to free the nerve. The problem with all this is that this explanation is not factually correct. Carpal Tunnels of this sort do occur, but they are rare, perhaps one in a hundred. I know this for a fact as I have treated many of them successfully and rarely even touch the Carpal Tunnel. It is a tragic misunderstanding leading to countless unnecessary, expensive and often unsuccessful surgeries.

True light was shed on this condition in 1973 when two researchers, Upton and McComas published what has become known as the "Double Crush Syndrome Hypothesis". They proposed that two lesser compressions on a nerve at different locations were additive and could have the same impact as one major compression, such as the Carpal Tunnel. This opened the possibility that compressions could occur anywhere along the course of a nerve, from the neck to the fingers. It turns out that it is not just compressions that are problematic, but nerve adhesions are even more so. Nerve adhesions are connective tissue growths attaching a nerve to the surrounding tissue, usually a muscle. These are very disruptive as they prevent the nerve from sliding as it is designed to do when the body is in motion. There is much research available supporting both these ideas. The problem then becomes finding where these adhesions and entrapments occur. This is done medically by a procedure called Electromyography which measures electrical activity of muscles by implanting needles and looking for decreased function. From the point of view of Applied Kinesiology this is expensive and cumbersome. Muscle Testing can accurately locate and correct these problems in much less time than it would take to set up the equipment to do the Electromyographic Testing.

In Lin's case, there were many dysfunctions present including muscle spasms, entrapments, adhesions, micro-evulsions of muscles, and subluxations of joints in the shoulder and neck. She was treated three times before all her symptoms disappeared. Not all Carpal Tunnels resolve this easily as there can be deep seated inflammation and metabolic problems contributing to the condition. However, nearly all these problems will resolve at a fraction of the cost of surgery and associated physical therapy.

Case #9 Shin Splints

Bill had developed painful muscle cramping in the lateral aspect of his left lower leg while hiking. The muscle that was cramping was the Tibialis Anterior, the muscle that flexes the foot upward. He wanted to know why and what to do to get rid of it. Almost always, these types of problems are best understood by looking for factors that interfere with the normal function of the involved muscle. We usually explore this by finding what else is wrong and trying to understand the pattern of dysfunction, rather than evaluating an isolated problem. They rarely occur alone. As we have illustrated in other cases, if there is no local damage to the tissues, it is useful to evaluate patterns of muscle function. This will often expose distal problems not otherwise obvious. In this case, there was no injury to the lower leg or knee. However, when we started testing the other muscles in his leg, the muscles connecting to his torso were also not functioning. His Rectus Femoris, the large muscle in the upper leg, was weak. Then we found a spastic muscle in his lower leg and a weak muscle in his upper leg. How are they related? We first tried to find what strengthens the weak Rectus Femoris. Muscle Testing revealed the entire abdomen was infected with bacteria. He had food poisoning and his only symptom was a shin splint in the left leg. Why would this happen?

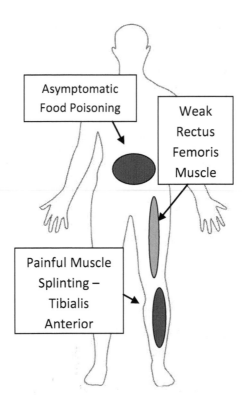

When we walk, at a certain phase of the gait, the right leg is extended backward. In this position, the muscle in the upper leg contracts to support the body at the same time the muscles behind the lower leg contract to push off for the next step. The food poisoning is inhibiting the Rectus Femoris, for the reasons we discussed, because the body does not want to contract the abdominal muscles to prevent compression of the infection. In this case, because the Rectus Femoris and the Gastrocnemius (the muscle in the calf) contract together, they are inhibited together. All muscles have a counterpart that opposes its function. For example, when you contract the Biceps Muscle in the front of the upper arm, the Triceps in the back part of the arm must relax. If not, they would fight each other. In this case, in the lower leg, the Gastrocnemius in the calf and the Tibialis in the shin area oppose each other. If the Gastrocnemius is inhibited, then the Tibialis Anterior will tend to spasm. This is what happened here. The solution to his shin splints was to treat the food poisoning. This released the inhibition of the muscles and allowed the shin muscles to function normally. Bill was given probiotics for the food poisoning and his shin splints disappeared in a few hours. I have seen similar cases to this many times.

Case #10   Reoccurring Blinking of the Left Eye

This is not exactly a pain, but an irritation. Jan had developed a reoccurring blink in the left eye, like a tic. There was no apparent reason, it had just started out of the blue a couple of days before and had become quite annoying. Like other irrational symptoms that pop up out of nowhere, we approached Jan's tic by exploring the body for other malfunctions to see what pattern it may be a part of. When I had her simply touch her eye, it did not cause a test muscle to go weak. But if I had her squeeze her eyes shut, it did. This indicates that the process of forcing the eyes closed is involved with a disturbed reflex. Rotating her head did not seem to affect the situation, nor did flexing or extending the head. What did affect the test muscle was challenging the stress patterns of the skull. Although the skull appears to be a solid stationary structure, it does in fact move ever so slightly, but enough to serve vital functions for the nerves that it supports.

With each breath the base of the skull flexes inward and the skull becomes slightly thinner and longer. With each exhale the opposite occurs with the sides of the skull flaring outward and the length of the skull becoming shorter. There is actually a side to side aspect of this motion also, and the process can become stuck in any phase of its motion. Sometimes cranial patterns will become distorted at birth and MRI studies of the skull show it to be distorted.

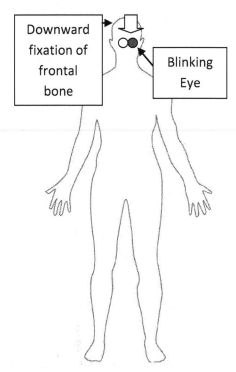

As with any joint in the body, positioning of joint patterns in the skull affects muscular patterns, facilitating some and inhibiting others. If an individual points his eyes upward, it will facilitate the neck extensors and also the extensor muscles in the back. At the same time, it will inhibit the muscles along the front of the neck and chest. If an individual looks down, the opposite will occur. In Jan's case her arm muscles weakend when she squinted, which does not tell us whether this is an upward looking pattern or a downward one, so we had to test. My guess was that it indicated a downward looking pattern because it was harder to squint and look up. When we tested by having her squint and flex with her head down her arm was still weak, but when she squinted and extended her head it got strong. What does this mean? Whenever we force a malpositioned joint into more malposition it will weaken the muscles of the body. Therefore, we know her skull was stuck in a downward flexion pattern. But which joints were involved? I had to test. When I pulled upward on her eye sockets to test and then rechecked the downward pattern, she was then strong. It was the frontal bone of her skull. I made several corrections to her skull and her eye blinking went away.

Case #11 Pain in a Baby

This case is interesting, not because it illustrates pain in a particular area of the body, but because it illustrates the power of Muscle Testing in interpreting odd behavior in a baby who could not speak to explain what was hurting. This young patient was sent to me by another doctor because he thought this infant was suffering from low back pain. The doctor thought this because the baby kept arching his back when picked up by his mother and held against her body. When I observed this behavior in my office it did appear the baby was suffering from back pain as he arched backwards with a grimace on his face, although he did not cry. However, when I tested the childs spine I could not find a problem. I then tested the child's organs and found his entire abdomen tested for bacterial infection. The baby had food poisoning! His arching backward was an attempt to get the pressure off his stomach when his mother was holding him. I prescribed several heavy doses of probiotics and by the next morning the arching behavior had stopped.

This is another area where Muscle Testing shines, in the evaluation of preverbal children and animals. To illustrate this with a couple of animal stories, a patient of mine brought me her dog who had recently become grossly overweight and had taken on a "hot dog" like appearance. The Vet wanted her to put him on a diet in spite of her protests that the dog's diet had not changed. When she brought him into the office after hours, our canine friend did have a "thick" swollen appearance. He muscle tested for parasites, specifically Trematodes. I gave her some herbs which she dutifully forced down his throat. She called me the next morning excitedly as the dog had shrunk back to normal size overnight. The "fat" was actually all water!

Another story, this same patient had a cat named "Harley" who was extremely sick. The Vet said he was dying of Kidney Failure and nothing could be done at this stage. When she brought Harley into the office he was indeed quite sick, staggering across the room like a drunk. I, of course, did not know if I could be of any help. Harley tested for a Mycoplasm infection in the kidney which explained why he had not responded to antibiotic intervention. Mycoplasms are cell wall deficient organisms and are notoriously resistant to antibiotics. I had her give him a tincture of herbs for Mycoplasms and another herb, Buchu leaves, which helps heal the kidneys. To our mutual amazement, Harley slowly recovered his health over the next few weeks. This is, but another example of the value of Muscle Testing.

Case #12   Non-Resolving Neck Spasm Following an Auto Accident

In treating whiplash injuries to the neck the usual course of treatment involves an initial inflammatory period of a couple of days to a few weeks. During this period the patient will have muscle spasms in the Para-cervical Musculature and inflammation in the joints that gradually declines. Therapy is centered around resolving inflammation and preventing scar tissue from restricting motion after healing. In a few patients the muscle spasm will not seem to resolve, even after the inflammation appears to be receding.

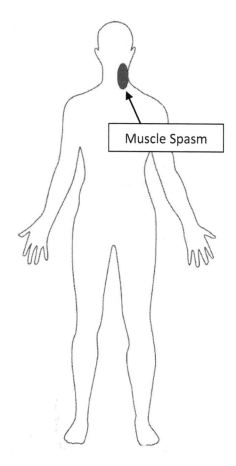

Muscle Spasm

For years I found these patients frustrating, and had trouble understanding why their progress stalled. A few years ago, I had such a patient named Linda. Although I did all the same things I do with other whiplash patients, she maintained a spastic condition on the left side of her neck. She was undergoing Physical Therapy, Acupuncture, Orthopedic care and Massage Therapy in addition to my efforts, yet her progress stalled.

Over the preceding few years I had been developing more understanding of shoulder problems and often insights from one area of the body will shed light on another. With shoulder problems, particularly if there is a history of trauma, there are often micro-evulsions of muscles that prevent stability and strength from being achieved with therapy. The tendons and muscles do not attach directly onto bone, but instead connect to the Periostium, a fibrous sheath surrounding the bone.

Between the Periostium and the bone there is a thin sheet of fluid. Crossing this gap are small fibrous "Sharpies Fibers" that connect the Periostium to the bone proper. In Micro-Evulsions some of these sharpies fibers break leaving a bubble of fluid and weakness to the attachment. These areas are usually acutely sore to palpation. I had eventually learned to treat these problems by precisely identifying the location of the evulsions with Muscle Testing, and then using compression to initiate healing. One day while working on Linda it occurred to me that I had not ever checked her neck for Evulsions, particularly of the Scalene Muscles on the anterior aspect of the neck. When I did I quickly identified several and initiated treatment of them as I would on a shoulder. To my surprise, on her following visit she reported a significant improvement. I realized I had been overlooking a significant factor in her recovery.

Normally a Micro Avulsion will inhibit the contraction of the muscle to prevent further tearing of the insertion. Why was I finding muscle spasm occurring in her neck if these were truly Evulsions? The answer, I believe, is that the muscles surrounding an Avulsion will spasm to shorten and relieve tension on the injured muscle. This helps to protect it. This is really a form of muscle splinting. When the Micro Avulsion is resolved the surrounding muscles relax as they have nothing to protect. Since treating Linda in this manner had produced such good results, I have incorporated this procedure in most whiplash cases and seen a marked success in their rate of improvement.

Case #13 Upper Back Pain Without Trauma

This is one of the most common complaints in a Chiropractic Office. "Doctor, I have a stabbing pain in my upper back and it is radiating up into my neck so I can hardly turn my neck." In almost all of these cases, the patient is talking about a rib head, the place where the ribs wrap around the body and attach to the spine. When ribs go out of place on the back they always become inflamed so any motion of the joint is painful. Very rarely, the patient will report some trauma that precipitated the pain, but it appears more frequently by itself without any identifiable cause. The one major cause where the structural component is dominant is when spinal curvature is present, a Scoliosis, and this is more common than you might think. Having said that, most cases of rib inflammation are not due to structural stress.

The Chinese recognized this long ago by noting that Acupuncture Points were often active at the rib joints and charted their significance for organ dysfunction. These are the Association Points mentioned earlier. In fact, the organs of the body are all represented in a row down the spine. The lung and heart points are in the upper back, and we do, in fact, find that there is usually a disturbance in these organs when the ribs in the upper back become painful.

While Scoliosis is usually regarded as primarily a structural problem with an unknown cause, I have noticed that in many cases there is an indication of lung or heart inflammation on the concave side. Applied Kinesiology Testing will often reveal an infection, which we might assume has been there a long time.

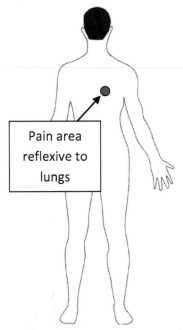

Pain area reflexive to lungs

These infections can be viral or bacterial, or more commonly parasitic. Many parasites are drawn to the lungs and sometimes the heart. Some, like the round worm Ascaris, breed in the lungs and have a life-cycle that cycles from the lungs to the intestinal tract and back again. It is common for the body to posture itself in relation to an inflamed organ by leaning over it. This has the function of reducing Fascial stress on the organ and allowing free pulsations, motion and blood circulation. So I suspect that this is a common cause of Scoliosis and thus rib pain.

So when Linda reported pain in her upper back, these were my thoughts. I had seen her before, so I knew she did not have Scoliosis. The next most likely thing to consider is infection, but it should be kept in mind that some people have an allergic inflammation of the chest organs or some other stressor, such as inflammation from air pollution. In Linda's case, Muscle Testing did indicate she had a lung infection, a virus. I have found that a large percent of lung infections are a metastasis from the intestinal tract, although an air borne infection is also possible. She did have an intestinal virus. Muscle Testing showed this was probably the same virus that she had in her lungs because they responded to each other through electromagnetic signals. Under these circumstances, it is best to treat the intestinal infection and wait for the lung infection to die out on its own. So I gave Linda Gamma Globulin supplements which quickly eradicated the intestinal virus, and I told her that the lung metastasis would fade away over the next day or so. I put a muscle stimulator on her inflamed rib to provide symptomatic relief until the infection went away.

The inflammation in her lung causing the Viscerosomatic response to her rib head was caused by free radical damage to the lung initiated by the virus. This will go away on its own as the viral infection fades, but it can be helped along by providing antioxidants to quell the irritating chemistry of the infection. I suggested she take a couple of large doses of Vitamin C. When taking antioxidants for an area of the body remote from the intestine, it is important to take a large dose all at once, rather than taking smaller doses over time. This is because if too little is taken the Vitamin C is used up by the tissues as it moves through the blood and will leave little for the lung inflammation at the end of the line. It is important to feed the tissues along with the whole course for the lungs, to still have enough left over to do the job. I have found the threshold dose to be about 2,000 mg and up in a single dose.

Case #14 Unresolved Hip Pain

Marcy is a young attractive woman in her late 20s. Three years earlier she had developed a pain in her left hip. She had been a long distance runner participating in marathons and tri-athlete events. There had been no trauma, but she had trouble with a gradually increasing pain in her left hip that seemed not well localized. It hurt in a broad area across her hip. She was well off financially and had used her resources to travel the country seeking help. This included numerous doctors including Chiropractors, Physical Therapists, Orthopedists, Oriental Medical Doctors and some of the best Sports Doctors in the country, according to her. She had MRIs, CAT Scans and X-Ray studies done and nothing showed of any significance, and none of her therapies had produced any results. Her hip pain was ruining her life and she had given up all sports activities.

When I examined her, the main functional disturbance I noticed was her inability to raise her left leg without great pain when she was in the supine position. She had very little strength in her leg, and I could push it down with one finger. This was clearly related to the central problem. But what was causing it? Her spine did not seem to be a factor and she did not exhibit joint dysfunction in her hips. Also, the reflexes from the abdomen, such as food poison, which are so common, also were negative. Her heart and lungs were strong and did not seem to be a factor.

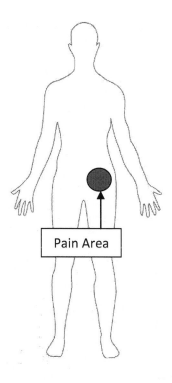

Pain Area

In these cases it is often instructive to very carefully examine the exact anatomical location of the pain. Although she described the pain over a broad area of the left hip and inguinal area, when I started Muscle Testing, the area that displayed a weakness was just anterior to the hip joint. It was quite sore to palpation. What was there? It turns out that the large muscle in the anterior leg, the Rectus Femoris, has two attachments; one just below the top of the hip and one right in front of the hip joint, right where it hurt. When I used my finger to support this attachment of the Rectus Femoris muscle in front of the hip joint, her leg muscle became instantly strong. I knew she was suffering from a Micro Avulsion strain of the Rectus muscle at this attachment.

I treated this strain with MyoFascial Rolfing Structural Integration Techniques, which took about one minute. When she got up from the table her pain was gone for the first time in years. She began to cry. She could not understand all the years of frustration, seen so many doctors and spent so much money on something that was so easy to fix. The answer is rooted in the nature of human perception. Doctors, like all of us, see what they are conditioned to see.

Case #15   Pain Raising the Left Leg

John experienced weakness raising the left leg and the leg flexors were weak when tested in a flexed position. There was also a general aching in the hip region when he tried to move his leg. This problem had started slowly and had gradually gotten worse. No trauma was involved. He could not sleep on that side anymore as it caused him to awaken in the night with aching in his hip. Usually these problems involve the Sacroiliac Joint on the same side and some abdominal irritation as the precipitating factor.

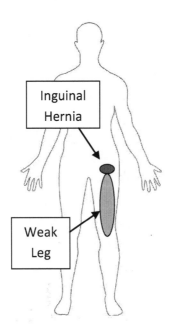

John's Sacroiliac Joint seemed fine and his intestines were clear of infection and were not sore to palpation. Sometimes intestinal infection will not show with straight Muscle Testing, but will show if the intestines are stretched in some direction while the Muscle Testing is being done. I began stretching the intestines in different directions while Muscle Testing. Nothing showed until, I got down near the Inguinal Ligament, the heavy fibrous band that suspends across the lower abdomen from the Pubic Symphesis to the Ilium. When I pulled my hand towards the ligament, he suddenly tested weak. If I pulled away from the ligament he got strong. But it was not an infection. There is a small canal here between the abdomen and the leg through which blood vessels enter the leg. Sometimes the intestines will start to balloon through this opening causing a Hernia. This was most probably an Incipient Inguinal Hernia. When I had the patient pull the Hernia upward, his leg went instantly strong.

What was happening here was that the contraction of the leg muscle on leg flexion also involved contraction of the abdominal muscles for support. This caused pressure downward and irritated the hernia. His body did not like this and inhibited the leg muscles as a protective mechanism. I had John lie on his side while I tractioned the fascia for the hernia away from under the inguinal ligament. When he stood up, his pain was gone and the muscles in his leg were strong. This kind of treatment will only work if the Hernia is small. Larger ones usually need medical intervention.

Case #16 Dropped Anterior Arch in the Right Foot

Bruce complained of pain in the anterior arch of the left foot. Usually in these cases you will find one of the joints at the ball of the foot sore to pressure, and that was the case here. We have

63

been treating cases like Bruce's by adjusting the involved joints and providing an anterior arch support in the shoe. This does help and will often relieve the inflammation.

However, it does not really address why the arch has dropped in the first place. I do not have a sure answer, but an observation. The anterior arch is the area in Foot Reflexology that is reflexive to the lungs. Foot Reflexologists will dig into these areas with their pointed little fingers as a way of treating the lung. I have noticed in patients with a dropped anterior arch, that there is often a problem with the lung on the same side. In Bruce's case, it was a parasite infection. I usually treat the lung problem, as I did in this case, but it did not seem to have any immediate effect on resolving the foot problem. My experience is that Anterior Arch Drop is a degenerate problem that takes time to correct, partly by supporting the foot with arches, partly by adjusting the joints, and partly by treating the underlying energetic problem in the lung.

Case #17 Restless Leg Syndrome

Sandra was a 60 year old woman who had been diagnosed with Restless Leg Syndrome. This is a condition where the leg muscles start to "crawl", often when resting or during sleep. This is a very uncomfortable condition. The medical profession has decided this problem is due to a Central Nervous System Disorder, akin to Parkinson's Disease and its associated tremors, and thus prescribes Sinemet, the Dopamine Neurotransmitter that is deficient in Parkinson's Disease. Research has shown this therapy is not very successful and needs to be constantly re-drugged with alternative drugs to hold the symptoms at bay. While it is possible a very small number of Restless Leg cases are of a Central Nervous System nature, there is very compelling reason to think that the vast majority of these cases are due to irritations of the Peripheral Nervous System, thus making the Sinemet therapy both unnecessary and dangerous.

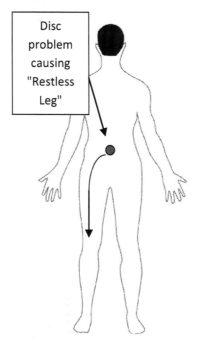

It is dangerous as the brain gradually becomes insensitive to the Dopamine, and thus requiring larger and larger doses until it will eventually not work at all. The problem with this is that Dopamine is essential to the brain, as any Parkinson's patient will tell you. I have written about the research supporting the Peripheral Nervous System Hypothesis elsewhere (see www.NaturalCureDoctor.com). Modern Chiropractic Technique in the form of Applied Kinesiology makes locating the source of the irritation quite easy, and thus opens the door to an often quick resolution of this condition without the use of drugs at all.

Although the nerve irritation can occur anywhere along the course of any of the major motor nerves, in Sarah's case the source of the irritation was a disc protrusion in her lower back. Her Neurologist who put her on the Sinemet did not check her for this problem, assuming without evaluation that the problem was in her brain. Upon examination in our office, the disc irritation became apparent. She had just run out of her Sinemet prescription so I asked her to wait a few days to see if treatment of her disc would reduce her symptoms enough to make the use of Sinemet unnecessary. She agreed to give it a try.

This patient was treated with traction on her back with a flexion traction table and almost immediately we began to see her symptoms abate. She started sleeping through the night. Further treatment over the next few weeks continued to reduce her symptoms to negligible levels.

Many of these cases that I have seen are due to adhesions on the motor nerves, which cause an irritation of the nerve and produce the resulting muscle "crawling." When this is the case, most of the time the symptoms can be eliminated in one visit, or at the most, two or three. I have never seen a case of Restless Leg Syndrome that did not respond to this kind of therapy. This illustrates the misconception regarding this automatically, as a Central Nervous System Disorder. I have discussed this at more length on my website www.NaturalCureDoctor.com.

Case #18 Acute Hip Pain with Sciatica

A number of years ago I took a trip to Costa Rica to vacation at a remote jungle resort. As the resort location is too distant from urban areas, the access to doctors is minimal.

Word quickly got out that an American doctor was visiting and I had a number of patients arrive asking for my help. One of them was a young woman in her 30s. She and her husband owned the wilderness resort next door to the one I was visiting. She had apparently developed a hip pain and Sciatica so bad they were planning on selling the resort as she could no longer do the work.

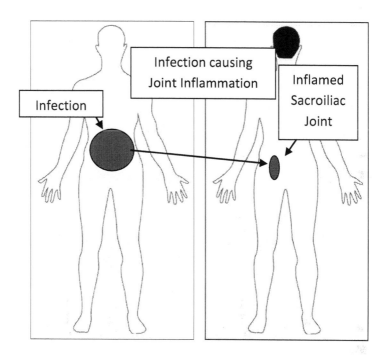

The resort I was staying at had set up a massage table out in the jungle so I could accommodate patients. It was an unusual clinic, with monkeys peering down at me from tree branches 100 feet in the air. This young American woman, we will call her June, arrived one day dragging her left leg behind her like a bird with a broken wing. She had been back to the US for evaluation and treatment, but had not benefited from what was done. I put her on the table and began using Applied Kinesiology to evaluate her condition. She could hardly raise her leg at all. Fortunately, I had brought a number of bottles of different herbs for myself, in case I became sick. I used these to test her and quickly realized she had an extensive Yeast Infection in her intestine. In fact, with the bottle on her abdomen she could raise her leg with much more ease. This indicates that this was correcting an important dysfunction in her leg and hip. As mentioned earlier, there is a Viscerosomatic reflex between an inflamed intestinal lining and the Sacroiliac Joint, often causing fluid build-up and inflammation in the joint. Her SI Joint was seriously inflamed and was the source of her Sciatic neuralgia.

I could not say that the Yeast Infection was her only problem because inflammation was so extensive that it interfered with Orthopedic Testing. However, in cases like this with a severe infection, I always treat the infection first. I was sorry I was leaving as I could not follow-up her case, but I gave her the herb for yeast infection that I had brought for myself and asked her to let me know how things turned out by email. When I arrived back home in the US two days later, I got an email from her telling me she had completely recovered. How amazing, this simple treatment restored her health and saved her resort.

This case illustrates how Viscerosomatic reflexes can mimic Orthopedic problems. Severe Sciatic neuralgia is almost always viewed as a low back problem involving a disc.

I had another similar case a couple of years before that. One of my relatives had been in a severe auto accident many years before and she had been seriously hurt. In fact, she was in a wheel chair for a while. She gradually recovered and all was well for a few years. Then her back started hurting again. It became worse and worse. She went to her doctors including her regular MD, her Acupuncturist, her Chiropractor, and her Massage Therapist. She was taken to the emergency ward several times for severe back pain. Her doctor had her on pain killers, muscle relaxers and sleeping pills. Her life was miserable. This had been going on for three years. Everyone assumed the problem was from her auto accident as the symptoms were so similar. She called me one day to tell me she was going to sell her horse ranch as she could not do the work anymore.

As a fluke, she came to visit shortly afterward and asked me to work on her back. The Muscle Testing quickly revealed she was suffering from simple bacterial food poisoning. I did not have any Acidophilus in the house, so I had Metagenics mail a bottle to her house. She called me the day after it arrived to tell me all her pain was gone. It has never returned. She did not sell her ranch.

Case #19   Chest Pain on Taking a Deep Breath

A man brought in his 10-year-old daughter Sandra to see if I could help with a chest pain she experienced while taking deep breaths. She had been diagnosed with Asthma several years before and had been on medication for it for years. The problem was the medication did not seem to be working anymore. She had not used the medication much for several months because it did not stop the pain. The pain seemed to be both in front and in the rib joints in the back, and only occurred at the end of the breath when she would breathe in.

I began Muscle Testing to see if anything showed up in her chest. This testing indicated a disturbance in her lungs on both sides. Some of the rib joints on her back were sore to palpation. Although she was diagnosed with Asthma, I checked her lungs for infection anyway in case something had been missed.

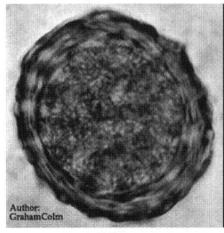 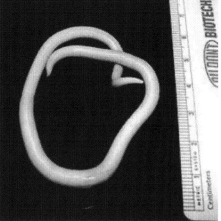

Fertile egg in human feces   An adult female Ascaris

In fact, she did test positive for a worm infection – Ascaris Lumbricoides. This little worm breeds in the lungs and will cause lung inflammation. I believe Sandra had been taking the wrong medication for years. She needed a worm solution, not Asthma medication. This was a subclinical infection, so I gave her herbs to help the body reject the infection.

Within three weeks all her chest pains had disappeared and have not returned. She did not have Asthma after all. I have seen worm infections mistaken for Asthma several times.

Case #20 Radiating Pain Down the Left Arm

Joan complained of a pain radiating down her left arm. The pain had been there for the last three weeks and did not appear to be getting better. It seemed to radiate from her upper back, but her neck was also painful and spastic. There was no trauma involved. She could not sleep well because the aching became worse at night.

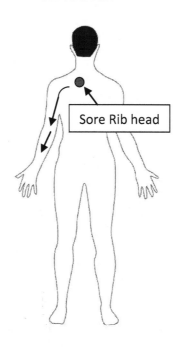

Sore Rib head

There were indications that she did have some degenerate problems in her neck. I had taken X-Rays previously which showed a mild problem at C5, but it did not seem enough to account for what she was going through. Her arm weakened when downward pressure was placed on her head, this is a test for cervical disc problems which could cause nerve pain in the arm. However, distracting the neck did not seem to improve her pain. Her neck needed treatment, but was not likely the cause of her problem.

Palpation revealed the rib joints in her upper back were sore and pressure on them did elicit pain down her arm. This is actually a common source of arm pain. When rib joints become inflamed and Subluxated they often irritate nerves in the arm, although there is no direct anatomical connection between the two. I do not know why this occurs, although hypothesize a connection within the spinal cord.

However, the underlying cause of the rib Subluxaton is another matter. Some of these problems are caused by curvature of the spine, Scoliosis. When the spine is twisted it pulls on the rib attachment to the spine causing inflammation. However, Scoliosis is not the most common cause of these problems. As noted earlier, the Association Points reflecting organ stresses are all located at these rib joints.

In the upper back, we most commonly see inflammation in the heart or lung being the underlying cause. When this is the case, it has been my experience that the rib problem will not go away with Chiropractic manipulation alone without correcting the underlying organ disturbance. In Joan's case, the problem was her heart, which tested for a Potassium deficiency. She was under stress. Often when an individual is under stress, the Adrenal Glands over the kidneys become hyperactive and use large amounts of Potassium.

When they are hyperactive they use up the available Potassium so it is not distributed in adequate amounts for the rest of the body. Potassium is the main intercellular mineral and is necessary for muscle function. The heart is the most active muscle in the body so it is the first to suffer. In this case, the Adrenal dysfunction needed attention to allow the heart muscle to get enough Potassium.

Adrenal Glands can rarely be normalized with nutrition alone, but need a quiet environment with deep sleep and calmness to rebuild, as well Potassium supplementation and Melatonin for rest. She returned to normal in a couple of weeks and her rib pain faded away.

Case #21 Shoulder Pain When Raising Right Arm

Debra was the wife of a doctor and came to see me because of a shoulder pain that had originally started twelve years prior when she hurt herself lifting weights. She had had X-Rays and an MRI of the shoulder which revealed only a minor injury to the rotator cuff, not enough to account for the dysfunction she was suffering from. She could not raise her arm without pain or reach behind her back to undo her bra. She had tried numerous types of therapy including several years of Physical Therapy and exercises, Acupuncture, Chiropractic, Deep Muscle Massage and even a Detoxification Program. Her doctor told her she was not a surgery candidate as nothing showed on the imaging studies. My experience with these types of cases is that many doctors fail in diagnostic accuracy because they are looking for a cause of the problem, such as a Sprained Ligament, a Cervical Subluxation or a Rotator Cuff tear. Sometimes one or more of these are found, but treatment for them does not resolve the problem. For the patient, this is often a bitter disappointment if surgery is unsuccessful given the greater costs and recovery time. The actual cause is a matrix of dysfunction and is exactly the type of problem that the disease model is so unable to respond to. This is because correcting one or a few of the problems will make no difference. The entire matrix of problems needs to be resolved and the benefits appear suddenly at the end of a whole series of corrections. After twelve years of care, you would think she would have done everything that could be done. Each practitioner had his idea of what was causing it and treated her accordingly. Yet it took only three treatments to return complete strength to her arm and another couple to return most of her range of motion. So what was wrong?

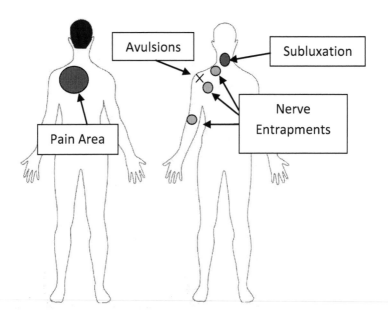

The answer was that she had about 30 smaller problems, each which took a few seconds to a half hour to correct. These included numerous nerve entrapments and nerve adhesions, where nerves become glued to the muscle fascia. She also had Subluxations in her shoulder joint and neck. She had two or three Micro-Avulsions of the Deltoid Muscle in her shoulder and she had Mycoplasmic infections in her shoulder joint and in the muscles over and around her shoulder blade. Infections are common in injured joints as the joint capsule is ruptured and the infections have easy access to the rich joint fluids where they breed so easily. These are difficult to locate using standard Orthopedic tests, but are very easy to identify with Chiropractic Applied Kinesiology.

Treatment is quite simple once the various dysfunctions are identified. It included adjusting of her neck and shoulder, compression of the Micro-Avulsions, and deep muscle release of the nerve adhesions. The subclinical infections were removed using herbs and Rife Technology. To her, it was magic after what she had been through.

Case #22 Tennis Elbow

Pat came to our clinic because she had Tennis Elbow, a painful condition that hurts the outer aspect of the elbow, named I assume, because individuals suffered from this due to swinging a tennis racket.

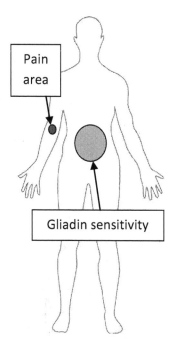

However, Pat did not play tennis. The assumption was that this condition was acquired from repetitive use of a computer mouse, as this requires constant use of the wrist extensor muscles that attach at the lateral aspect of the elbow, right where she had pain. This is not an unreasonable assumption, as use of any part of the body can cause wear and tear, and too much use will not allow proper repair. However, as you must suspect, there is more to the story.

One thing notable about this location for pain is that it is also the location of a major acupuncture point, the Large Intestine 11. Just as a precaution it is worth examining the Large Intestine and its associated Meridian, the Lung, to see if there is an organic contribution to this problem. She did report that she had been suffering from digestive disturbances as long as she could remember. To make a long story short, we sent in a lab test to check for Gliadin sensitivity which came back positive. Gliadin is a component of Gluten, a substance found in certain foods such as wheat. Some people have a genetic allergy to this which will cause digestive disturbances whenever it is encountered. It cannot be cured, only avoided. In Pat's case, she was forced to eliminate Gliadin containing foods which solved her digestive problems.

However, many people have Gliadin sensitivity who do not have tennis elbow. So we may assume, that by itself, this is not sufficient cause of her problem. I have treated many of these problems and see the same precipitating factors over and over. Tennis elbow has the same underlying cause as Carpal Tunnel.

Tennis Elbow is an inflammation of the insertion of the extensor muscles of the forearm. Like other Chiropractic problems, we begin our examination by investigating inhibition of the entire chain of extensor muscles from the hand to the neck. In all these cases we find variations on the same theme, entrapments of the nerves down the arm, Subluxations of the shoulder, elbow, neck, and other related disturbances. When these were corrected her problem faded away as they have on many similar patients before her. Tennis Elbow problems usually involve a series of treatments due to the inflammatory nature of the condition. The pain at the elbow is due to a Micro-Avulsion of the extensor muscles and their attachment, and needs to be compressed over and over to allow reattachment to occur. The length of the treatment is usually determined by the degree of Avulsion and inflammation.

Case #23 Aching Shoulder

A mother brought in her 10-year-old daughter who had been complaining of pain and aching in her left shoulder. It seemed to bother her most at night. There was no traumatic injury. When it came to identifying specifically what hurt her, things became increasingly vague. It seemed to hurt her somewhere in her shoulder blade, but over a general area. She could move her arm well, but she felt more discomfort when she raised it above her head. The shoulder flexors and Deltoid Muscle tested weak. There were no sore places in the tendon and ligament and Rotator Cuff. What could this be?

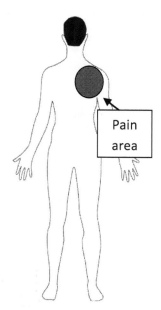

Usually in these cases, the underlying problem is reflected in some muscle weakness. Since her shoulder flexors tested weak I decided to use this to test for what is wrong. I checked for nerve entrapments and did find two which I corrected, but this did not ease her pain or strengthen the shoulder flexors. Putting traction on the neck did not have any effect. However, when I pushed laterally on her neck and the muscle did strengthen. Finally, some positive indication! I palpated her neck and found considerable spasm on one side. It appears on investigation that the neck was simply Subluxated, so I asked if I could adjust her neck. When I did the audible release was unusually loud. She stared up at me with a serious look on her face and let out a big "Wow!" Then a big smile slowly grew across her face and she said excitedly, "My pain is gone!" Again, it was not a shoulder problem at all, it was her neck.

Case #24 Severe Sciatica

A young Indonesian woman was brought into my clinic in a wheelchair. She had developed severe Sciatic pain a few months before with radiating pain down the left leg. There was no precipitating trauma. It just started one day and got worse and worse until she was in pain 24 hours a day and had become bedridden.

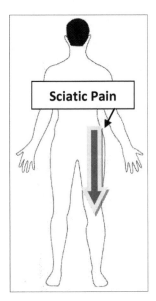

She had been evaluated by an Orthopedist and a Neurologist at a local hospital, including X-Rays and an MRI. Nothing showed on the imaging so she was sent to Physical Therapy for three months at three times a week with no improvement in her condition. At that point, the hospital informed her that there was nothing wrong with her and discontinued treatment, a sure sign her insurance had run out.

She was in so much pain that it took three people five minutes to move her from the wheel chair to the Chiropractic table for examination. Every slightest motion caused her to cry out in pain. There was something irritating her Sciatic Nerve which had become severely inflamed, but where was the irritation located? The hospital had already looked for disc problems and found none. The nerve did not test for infection. I decided to test for the irritant by using a simple technique I developed myself years before, I called it "Nerve Brushing." I had noticed that tapping or brushing the skin over a nerve would weaken any muscle I was testing, only if the nerve was irritated. If the nerve was not irritated this did not occur. This allowed me to easily locate the irritant by brushing in a sequence of short brushes up the length of the nerve until the arm muscle being tested suddenly strengthened. The irritant could be assumed to be located between the strong and weak responses along the length of the nerve. In this woman's case, the muscle remained weak until I reached her buttock when it suddenly became strong.

I know that a common cause of Sciatic Nerve irritation is the Pyriformis Muscle that runs horizontally from the sacrum to the hip. The Sciatic Nerve is known to either pass right through the belly of the muscle, or to pass under it. In either case, if the muscle becomes too contracted it can compress the nerve. When I palpated the Pyriformis Muscle, it was spastic and very painful. I guessed at this point, that she had what is known as a "Pyriformis Syndrome", a spastic Pyriformis Muscle with a compressed and irritated Sciatic Nerve under it. I put her on her side carefully, and after warning her that it might hurt a little, I did a deep Fascial stretch of the muscle. She nearly levitated off the table in pain and let out a scream, yet within two minutes was able to get back into her wheel chair without any help. I knew I was on the right track. After two more treatments she came into the clinic walking on her own. In three more treatments she had recovered.

This case shows the great value of Muscle Testing in simplifying diagnosis. The hospital had spent thousands of dollars and months of time, and had not figured out what was wrong. I had spent five minutes and had already started correcting the problem - Thank you Dr. Goodheart!

Chapter - 4

Chiropractic, Systemic Imbalance and Infection

For many years, I was not aware of the pervasive presence of subliminal infection and treated the manifestation of their activities as nutritional problems, toxic states, Adrenal insufficiency, MyoFascial displays and Subluxations. Acute infections are the domain of Medical Doctors as this is one of their specialties and antibiotic treatment is usually so effective.

However, due to the use of antibiotics in farming as well as overuse of antibiotic prescriptions, many microbes are becoming increasingly resistant to medical treatment. This is especially dangerous as the public is conditioned to have faith in antibiotics, and thus are unaware that these drugs are becoming increasingly ineffective. This faith that modern medicine and antibiotics will solve infectious problems has translated into a public apathy about addressing this growing risk of resistant bacteria. It is played out in a lack of political will to keep the environment cleaner to reduce exposure, and to better control antibiotic use in medicine and farming. This psychology is not just a risk factor for acute infection, but creates an environment in which low grade exposure to microbes and a gradual accumulation of subliminal infections is becoming commonplace. This exposure to microbes, combined with other factors that reduce immune resistance can be a major contributor to gradually declining health and health longevity. These factors include things like poor food quality, toxins and a stressful lifestyle. In my practice new patients often ascribe their pains to many different causes other than this, and are often surprised to find their health recovering when treated for infection. This includes treatment for many traditional Chiropractic problems such as stiff neck, low back pain and sometimes Sciatica.

It takes much longer to resolve these problems if the underlying infections are not addressed. Even with the intention to clear infections, we do not have the technology to either find all infections or clear them if found. This is an obvious state of affairs with conditions like Aids, Chronic Fatigue and Lymes Disease, but the persistence of chronic infection may be more common than we suppose. Take Herpes Infection as an example, which is believed to infect nearly everyone. In these circumstances what we can do is build the immune system, which has been dealing with these problems since the origins of life. There are theories of sexual reproduction proposing that sex is a biological mechanism to rid each generation of its microbial load. However, as we live longer and longer we will have to deal more directly with covert infections.

I believe Natural Healing can provide a better option to deal with many common infections like flu or common intestinal microbes without the risks associated with antibiotic use. These alternatives could help reduce antibiotic use. It is worth keeping in mind that, even with their correct use, antibiotics may damage Mitochondria and our health. Mitochondria are the organelles in cells that produce energy. It has been proposed that Mitochondria are actually bacteria and that, in our Phylogenetic past, became incorporated into cells in a permanent symbiotic relationship. This is thought to be true because Mitochondria looks like bacteria plus they have their own DNA which is passed down solely through the female side, and is not part of the nuclear DNA. If they are bacteria, they may as well be susceptible to degradation by antibiotics. Another concern is that antibiotic use frequently causes good bacteria to die in the intestinal tract and is followed by a surge of Fungal Infections to fill in the vacuum. The Intestinal Yeast can invade the body and cause other serious problems.

Throat Flu and Artificial Heat Treatment - Hot Air Therapy

One example, of non-antibiotic Natural Care for Flu is through the use of hot air. This is an important option to be aware of as Flu is Viral, not Bacterial, and does not respond to antibiotics anyway. Hot air works on viruses because it mimics the body's own response to Flu by making a fever. Viruses do not breed well in a hot environment, and do breed well in a colder environment. This is why so many people get sick when the weather turns cold. In fact, the infection usually starts in the back of the throat where the cold air hits before turning downward to the Lungs. This differentially cools this spot making it more susceptible to breeding Flu Viruses. The body will not make a fever until the infection spreads extensively in the body. When the infection spreads it becomes more dangerous because fever makes the body function much less efficiently. Fever takes energy from other vital metabolic activities to burn as heat, and in so doing reduces all survival functions except the immediate task of beating the Virus. Taking energy from other body functions makes you feel sick. This sickness from fever can sometimes be suspended by sitting in a very hot room, say 100 degrees Fahrenheit, so the extra heat needed to fight the infection is provided externally. Many times under these conditions the sense of being sick will completely disappear but reappear within a few minutes of leaving the heated environment. Sick people naturally gravitate towards heat for this reason. We can use this insight to our advantage by providing heat early in the infection cycle, before the fever stage is reached. This short circuits the need for advancing to fever and disadvantages the virus by blocking its breeding and allowing the immune system to eradicate it sooner.

People often ask me if getting into a sauna will do the same thing. The answer is "not usually." The reason for this is that the sauna will heat the whole body limiting the time you can stay heated to 20 to 30 minutes.

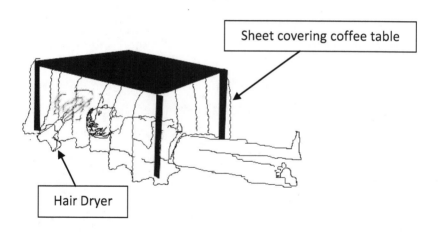

Sheet covering coffee table

Hair Dryer

This is not enough to eradicate the infection. Often it is necessary to sleep over night in a high heat environment to win. The length of time necessary is dependent on whether the body already knows how to beat the infection, or whether it is completely new. When the body responds to a new infection the white blood cells set out developing an antibody to kill the infection. An Antibody is a chemical secretion made by white blood cells that is specific for neutralizing a particular Antigen (an immune irritant – in this case the virus). This may take time.

Until it solves this problem of creating the correct antibody for the virus, the infection has the advantage and can spread rapidly. This is where the hot air comes in. It can block the viral breeding until the body learns how to make the appropriate antibody. A setup under a coffee table with a sheet and hair dryer, as illustrated above works fairly well. The part of your body sticking out from under the sheet can cool you down if you need it. You only need the heat where the infection is.

This heat treatment for infection can sometimes work even with severe infections. A number of years ago a young very concerned woman came to my office. She had been diagnosed with an infection in the back part of her skull, an Osteomyelitis. She had already been through several long episodes of antibiotic therapy and it had not affected the infection. Her doctors were proposing that, since the antibiotic therapy was not working, they cut away the back part of her skull and replace it with a metal plate.

Understandably she was somewhat hesitant to go along with this plan. She had ended up in my office to find out if alternative medicine had any solutions to her problem. After examining her and thinking about it, I started telling her about the role fever can play in eradicating infection and described the concept of creating an artificial fever. The infection was right near the surface of the body so it would be easy to heat with an external source. I recommended that she go home and put a heating pad on the back of her head continuously for three days then return for reevaluation. Just putting heat on an infection may not always be a wise thing to do, but in this case the inflammation from the infection was minimal, having the quality of a "cold infection." I felt it was worth a try. After the second day her infection completely disappeared and did not return. She was beside herself with joy!

Chiropractic Manipulation and Infection

Chiropractors have always maintained that spinal manipulation will positively influence the immune system. I had an experience in Chiropractic School that has given this idea some prominence in my mind. I was in an adjusting class and a student was using my neck to learn, and in the process threw my neck out of adjustment badly. Within a few minutes my head and throat became congested. It got steadily worse and within an hour I was at home in bed running a fever. It took about ten days to recover including getting adjusted by an experienced Chiropractor. Since then I think it is a good idea to keep the spine adjusted, by an experienced doctor, for general health reasons. With Applied Kinesiology it is easy to demonstrate that spinal manipulation can affect any part of the body.

Chapter - 5

Usable Concepts for Health

Longevity and Health

In terms of a real philosophy of health, the approach which forms the dominant paradigm in Western culture, of opposing disease using drugs and surgery, seems inadequate to address the needs of high performance health. Interestingly and sadly, Medical Doctors are one of the shortest living professions. According to the Indian Medical Association, Medical Doctors have a life span ten years shorter than their patients. You would think the Medical Doctors themselves would be concerned about this. Also statistics presented by Ralph Nader showing 100,000 to 150,000 yearly deaths in the US from this form of treatment should also warn the rest of us of the limits of Allopathic Medicine. They primarily attack disease using means foreign to normal health processes. Much of modern medicine is emergency medicine and serves well in that function. But this philosophy has its limitations. Athletes, for example, cannot rely only on the allopathic approach, in part because some drugs are illegal for them, but also because most drugs are damaging to the body with prolonged use and will interfere with their performance. The concept behind most drug use is to block the collapse of the body, but not to provide high performance.

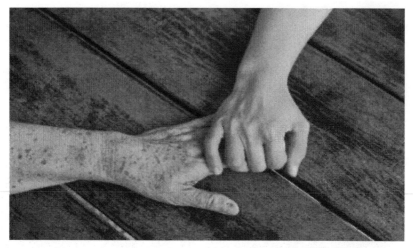

Image by FreeDigitalPhotos.net

High performance approaches to health are not just for athletes. Maintaining the biological system in a peak state leaves little room for disease, thus eliminating much of the role of modern drug medicine. The health discipline that encapsulates all the necessary thought for a practical approach to health is that of Longevity. As Dr. Wolford has noted, most factors that increase lifespan also decrease disease, prevent degenerate illness, and increase health and happiness.

Factors that influence longevity include everything that affects life. While you die from your weakest link, each factor contributes something to longevity and interacts with the others. However, some factors are more local or limited in their reach and some are systemic. This is a partial list of factors influencing longevity. We will discuss a few of them.

1. Antioxidant Status
2. Vitamins, Minerals, and Amino Acid Status
3. Recovery from Trauma
4. Spinal Health and Degeneration
5. Sexual Vitality
6. MyoFascial Problems
7. Psychological Health/Addictions
8. Sugar Metabolism
9. Glycation
10. Beauty
11. Balance and Proprioception
12. Exercise and Muscle Mass
13. Subclinical Infection and Immune Status (Pathogen Load)
14. Allergy
15. Digestion
16. Abdominal Health and Fiber
17. Mitochondrial Energy Production
18. Neurotransmitters/ Preventing Brain Degeneration
19. Toxicity and Detoxification
20. Chronic Inflammation
21. Cardiovascular Health
22. Telomere Length and Genetic Damage
23. Longevity Intelligence
24. Sleep
25. Stress
26. Zippity Doo Dah

Sexual Vitality

Everyone knows sex is wonderful and emotionally fulfilling. Yet, it is less obvious that we exist like salmon, to breed and die. Our DNA seems to care about supporting our existence only for sex, and when it sees that the game is over it will abandon us and stop supporting our life functions. Note the transformations of the years past menopause. I have been told by women that they lost their youthful appearance within one year of their cycles ending, although for others it can take much longer. Our DNA monitors our sexual excitement, anthropomorphically speaking. This depends on our hormones and vascular health and numerous other functions. We will talk about a couple of them here briefly.

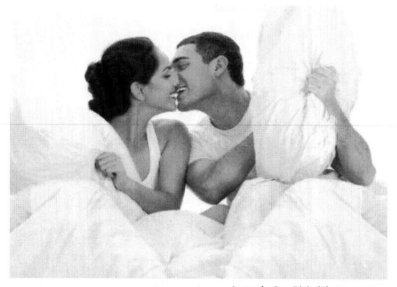

Image by FreeDigitalPhotos.net

I believe it is not possible to maintain youth without mimicking the physiological patterns of youth. All young sexually active people are flush with hormones. There is as much question about replacing hormones in pre-menopausal and post-menopausal men and women as there is recent research on artificial hormones suggesting an increased risk of cancer.

I will state first of all that these questions have not been completely answered, but as in many health decisions, we must proceed with the information that we have and what our instincts tell us we should do. We should also be aware that most of the information scaring us about cancer comes from pharmaceutical hormones, not bio-identical hormones. That is to say, horse Estrogens, Progestins and other modified hormones that are not normal to the human body.

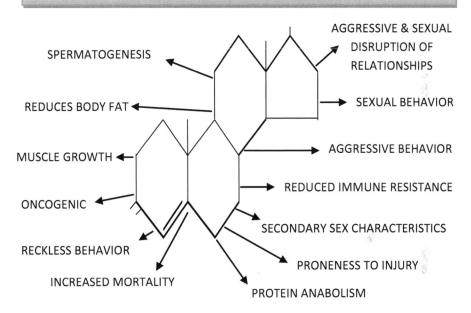

There have been many false deductions made from artificial hormones that have been applied to bio-identical hormones. This is not logical as they are completely different substances, although they are both referred to as hormones, as though they were comparable.

For example, it is known that some bio-identical hormones have opposite effects to artificial hormones in increasing risk for Cancer. Note natural Progesterone, which is Cancer-preventive versus artificial Progestins which are frankly carcinogenic. However, intuitively, there is still uneasiness. In part this concern is amplified by overemphasizing hormones and ignoring the context they occur in. For example, hormones tend to occur in opposing pairs so that, for example, Estrogen is buffered by Progesterone. The potency of Estradiol, the most potent Estrogen, is buffered by the concentration of Estriol, the weakest Estrogen that uses the same receptor sites as Estradiol. Estradiol itself, as it is metabolized, forms hyper Estrogens, Catechol Estrogens. What if these metabolites are controlled, how does this affect the carcinogenicity of hormone replacement? Rationally we would expect a reduction of toxic Estrogen metabolites to help. At the very least, all these factors need consideration. There are also other factors that affect carcinogenicity such as alkalinity of the body, Selenium and other nutrients, toxins and other such things. You simply cannot draw conclusions without a reasonable evaluation of these factors as they are interactive. So my guess is that hormone replacement may not be nearly as dangerous if the entire pattern of youthful physiology is upgraded, instead of just dropping an artificial hormone into an old person. I believe it is wise to proceed with replacing missing hormones to reestablish the patterns of youth, unless of course, Cancer is known to be present. We know what happens when we don't replace declining hormones. I respect anyone who makes a different choice under these circumstances, but I personally feel hormone replacement is essential.

Having said this there is a tendency by doctors to replace the final hormones in the steroid pathways such as Testosterone and Estradiol, and ignore the precursor hormones such as Pregnenalone and DHEA which make the other steroid hormones. As athletes know who use Testosterone, this hormone has many dangers including suppression of the testes and hormone production. Use of the precursor hormones does not normally do this, which is why they are not regulated. Studies measuring Testosterone levels with long term DHEA use does not support the idea that it raises Testosterone levels, which is probably why Testosterone itself is used to increase Testosterone levels. However, if the breakdown products of Testosterone are measured for an hour or three after DHEA ingestion, these metabolites rise sharply indicating that Testosterone was produced and metabolized. This suggests that taking smaller doses of DHEA more frequently may provide much of the Testosterone that is needed and provide a safer road.

While I am aware that Testosterone is usually regarded as the hormone that induces sexual desire, research does not support this statistically. Although there are wide human differences, in general, research shows the sex drive comes from Leutenizing Hormone and Follicle Stimulating Hormone, not Testosterone, although Testosterone is an essential ingredient. So sex drive for many people, cannot be turned on by only taking Testosterone, but likely involves actual sexual stimulation and probably Neurotransmitter status. Some Neurotransmitters are known to affect sex drive, such as Dopamine and Epinephrine. The latter is affected by Yohimbe, an aphrodisiac herb.

Another related factor is the capacity of the vascular system to respond to sexual excitement. We all know that Viagra has had a big impact on this problem, but does not solve the underlying problem of why Viagra is needed at all. This has much to do with the production of Nitric Oxide which is secreted by the Endothelial cells along the inside layer of the arterial system. It is known that taking DHEA with Pycnogenol, a pine bark antioxidant, can help restore this function. This suggests that the loss of Nitric Oxide may be due to free radical damage of the Endothelial Lining. Protecting the vascular system from this damage must be a part of preventing aging of the sexual system.

Antioxidant Status

In 1956, Dr. Denham Harman proposed the free radical theory of aging with his publication in the Journal of Gerontology. Most theorists concerned with aging accept some version of this idea and it is most probably wise to give this idea careful consideration. The basic idea here is that electron hungry molecules within the body originating from normal metabolism, toxins, infections etc. steal electrons from other chemical processes going on in the body causing their degradation. This degradation causes inflammation, inefficiency and aging. It is easy to imagine how this process could be a primary cause of problems in the body.

The free radicals set loose in the body are absorbed by antioxidants; substances such as Vitamin E, C, Selenium, Proanthocyanids, Vitamin A, Beta-Carotene, Glutathion etc., which donate electrons to neutralize free radicals, bringing this process to a halt. We would logically deduce that a shortage of antioxidants would allow this process to run unchecked within the body, like a wrecking crew, until we succumb to the damage. Most people concerned with nutrition that I know believe that free radicals are an underlying cause of disease formation and shorten youthspan. It is known, for example, that longevity is positively correlated with Glutathione levels in the body. There are countless studies showing the benefits of antioxidants on various systems of the body.

The other side of free radical control is to limit the production of free radicals in the first place, rather than quelling them after they have formed. Many aspects of life that cause free radical production are under our control. For example, this can be done by keeping sun exposure down to prevent sunburn, reducing toxic exposure or controlling infection, to name a couple.

Keeping the Spine Young

As a Chiropractor, an area of special interest is helping my patients maintain a healthy spine. It is hard to deny the far reaching negative effects on health and well being of an aging and degenerating spine. An old spine is stiff and painful and can produce paralyzing pain when nerves become compressed. This area of health has been championed by the Chiropractic profession and, as a central concept of health, has been under attack by the medical profession since its conception by D. D. Palmer a hundred years ago. It is first worth noting that the Chiropractic field is not one monolithic viewpoint, but is a field with great diversity.

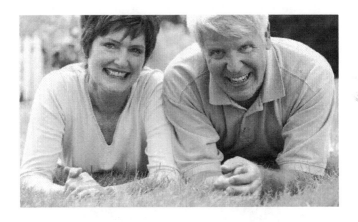

Branches of Chiropractic, such as Applied Kinesiology that interface closely with the ideas of Naturopathic Medicine and Basic Medical Science, take into account the full complexity of the body and its relation to the spine. Traditional Chiropractic has always emphasized the outflow of nerves from the spine and the interference of these nerves as a causal factor in disease. In fact, the nerves go both ways and the status of the spine is intimately related to the condition of the rest of the body.

Chiropractors have emphasized the effect of Subluxations on spinal degeneration. Subluxations are malpositions of vertebrae that induce nerve interference. As I have mentioned earlier, I believe these are of two major types; Traumatic and Reflexive. All types of Subluxations can cause inflammation and thus have the potential for causing deterioration of the inflamed tissues. By far the worst of these two for causing degeneration is traumatic Subluxation. Once degeneration is set in motion is seems to be a progressive phenomena advancing through several identifiable stages. What can be done to prevent it or reverse it once it has started?

A general characteristic of Subluxated joints is a lack of motion, or fixation of the joint. This lack of motion starves the connective tissue, such as discs. This occurs because they have no blood supply and eat like a sponge through the diffusion of nutrients to the cells. This diffusion depends on motion. Knowing this, Chiropractors have always emphasized re-establishing motion in fixated joints with spinal manipulation.

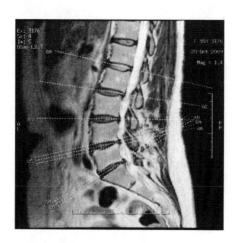

I have seen many X-Rays in Chiropractic offices of spines that have been repeatedly adjusted over time that showed positive regeneration of discs. What percentage of cases respond to this treatment I do not know, but it does happen. Based on this, I believe the advice to get regular spinal Chiropractic care is sound. More advanced degeneration and protrusions of spinal discs can be better treated using a new technology called Non-Surgical Spinal Decompression.

I have had one of these machines in my office for about five years and can testify that we have had over 90 percent success in treating these conditions. It is so successful that most spinal surgeries are now outdated.

Infection

Nearly all of us carry low grade infections that we are unaware of. We are used to thinking of infections as something that make us sick. Often, when I tell patients they have food poisoning, they respond with a comment that goes something like - "How could I have food poisoning when I feel fine?"

I have to demonstrate the effects on their muscular system or sore Alarm Points, before they will take me seriously. This is the tip of the iceberg. It is probably not possible to get all infections out of the body. They quietly destroy joints, kill organs, weaken our bodies and create Cancer, all without many indications that this is occurring at all.

I have sent patients back to their Medical Doctor to be treated for an infection, only to have the good doctor inform them that they did not have an infection and refuse treatment.

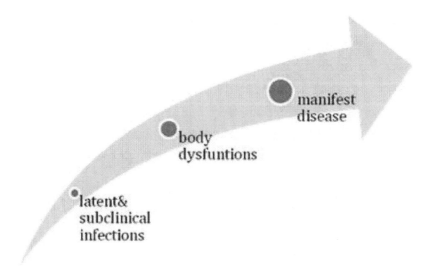

The reason why this happens is that the feedback for infections is so poor that doctors cannot agree whether there is an infection present or not. I am convinced from years of experience that standard lab testing, while vital, is very limited in its ability to expose covert infections. The reason why I feel this way is based on a number of observations. First, many lab tests do not agree with each other, thus exposing their limited detection abilities. You would think the answer is to order as many tests as possible, but this is unrealistic due to cost and the trouble doing all the tests.

Therefore, many doctors run one major test and make their judgment based on the results of this test. They sometimes believe the single test, even if there are other clinical signs of infection. We can be sure that conventional laboratory testing does not have a perfect correlation with actual clinical infections. Many years ago I used to date a woman who was the sole lab technician in a hospital in Tacoma, Washington. One day I asked her what the difference was in how the older, more experienced doctors utilized her in comparison to the new inexperienced doctors.

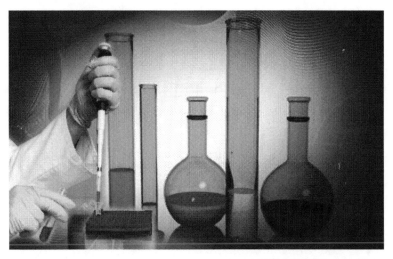

We place great value on lab testing for infections, yet it is marginally effective for finding covert infections.

Her answer surprised me. She said, "The experienced doctors either did not request testing at all, or only ordered single tests. Young inexperienced doctors ordered whole panels of tests." If nothing else, this statement is a commentary on the relative value of clinical observation and what can be observed through direct experience, verses information from laboratory testing.

A second observation is that some tests pick up many more infections than others. Quite commonly, Dermal Skin Testing will pick up ten times as many infections as Stool Testing. But can we assume that Dermal Testing will find them all? Not much chance of that.

We also have other forms of testing, we might term them "New Age Tests" because they utilize newer technologies, but more than that they are suggestive in nature, not definitive in nature. These include Applied Kinesiology Muscle Testing, O-Ring Testing, Voll

Testing and LSA Testing (the latter two are new technologies which use Electro-Diagnostic Testing) as well as others, potentially. However, what they lack in specificity they gain in sensitivity, speed and cost. Most doctors who use these forms of testing have had the experience of seeing positive therapeutic results based on their use when conventional testing failed. This has happened countless times in my clinic. If we put the uncertainty about both Conventional and New Age Testing up front in our minds, then it makes most sense to use conventional testing first in the most serious clinical conditions because the consequences of uncertainty can be fatal. In less serious conditions, or ones that develop slowly, it makes more sense to use "New Age Tests" because it is so sensitive, inexpensive and fast. Where needed, Conventional Testing could be used to confirm results of New Age Testing, to increase their level of certainty. This is a more directed use of lab testing, which is much more cost effective than using them for screening. When Conventional Testing is used for screening many come back negative. This is grossly inefficient, given other options available, and greatly increases the cost of evaluation.

Regardless of the testing method used, our goal should be to identify infections that are degrading some aspect of our body, and weed them out until they have very minimal effects, then, keep our guard up to watch for new developments.

As I mentioned earlier, the incidence of infection has increased hundred-fold in my practice in the last ten years. Most of these infections are not recognized as such. This is true, in part, because some of these infections were not common to this part of the world and doctors are not used to recognizing or treating them. This is especially true of parasite infections. I mean this in the narrow sense of the word to include tape worms, round worms and flat worms or flukes and Protozoal infections. These were present all along, but the increased incidence is alarming. I believe we can expect an increase in degenerative and chronic disease as a result. Flat worms, along with Mycoplasmic and Fungal Infections, seem attracted to eating and inhabiting connective tissue and I suspect contribute to such problems as Varicose Veins, Aneurysms, Prolapsed Organs, Arthritis, Hernias and possibly Strokes. They also are an underlying cause of pain and are reflected into the Musculoskeletal system causing many Chiropractic problems.

Exercise

This has so many benefits that it would take a book to do any justice to the topic. We all know that it can build cardiovascular health and build muscle. There are a number of specific effects that exercise has that are worth knowing about.

Exercise has a major effect on your hormones. When you start doing resistance exercising both Growth Hormone and Cortisol begin to rise together, but Growth Hormone rises faster as you see in the chart below. This fact has great consequences for the health outcome of exercise. The peak of Growth Hormone is within 30 minutes after exercise is started. Growth Hormone is Anabolic, meaning it adds protein and muscle to the body. As long as it is dominant we would expect the body to become stronger. If exercise is continued much beyond the half hour mark Cortisol rises above Growth Hormone. Cortisol is catabolic, meaning it breaks the protein in the body down. This is where continuing exercise past the half hour mark can become a detriment to the body.

The more intense the exercise the more likely it is to release Growth Hormone. This hormone is actually released mostly at peak intensity, so short bursts of intense exercise will provide more positive results than a long drawn out slower exercise workout.

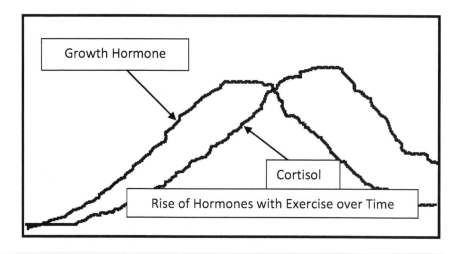

Growth Hormone

Cortisol

Rise of Hormones with Exercise over Time

Recent research has provided evidence that short intense exercise also helps preserve Telomeres, terminal chains of DNA that shorten each time a cell divides and are associated with preserving youth.

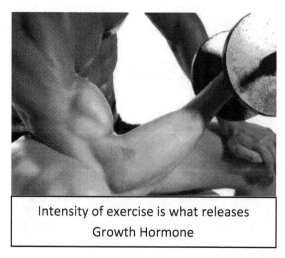

Intensity of exercise is what releases
Growth Hormone

Another great benefit of exercise is the release of Nitric Oxide, a substance produced by the inner epithelial lining of the arteries.

Nitric Oxide causes vasodilatation of the arteries and capillaries; in fact vasodilatation will not occur without it. One major cause of ED (Erectile Dysfunction) is a low production of Nitric Oxide. Nitric Oxide also plays a role in clearing plaque from the inner lining of the arteries and thus helps prevent Cardio-Vascular Disease. However, Nitric Oxide is also very aggressive chemically and functions as a Free Radical creator. For this reason it works best when it is released in the body in flushes, rather than keeping it as a continuously high level. One problem with the drug Viagra is that it keeps Nitric Oxide high for too long and this is the probable cause of vision loss in men taking it. The free radicals damage the eyes. On the other hand, this artery cleansing effect occurs best with higher levels of Nitric Oxide, thus this beneficial effect would be gained during exercise or sex.

MyoFascial Problems

This is an area of health and dysfunction that has almost completely escaped the awareness of conventional medicine. The result of this oversight has been a tragic misapplication of dangerous and damaging therapies to otherwise simple problems. Examples of this are surgeries for Carpal Tunnel pain and the use of Sinamet (a Dopamine drug) to treat Restless Leg Syndrome. Both of these problems are most commonly the result of MyoFascial Dysfunction and are treated inappropriately due to miscomprehension of the true nature of the symptoms.

Fascia is connective tissue that occurs in sheets throughout the body and surrounds virtually every tissue and organ. Fascia that surrounds muscle is called the Epimysium. Fascia that surrounds nerves is called the Epineurium. It also surrounds all organs. Fascia is continuous throughout the body. There is only one fascia. It serves different functions.

Nerve Structure

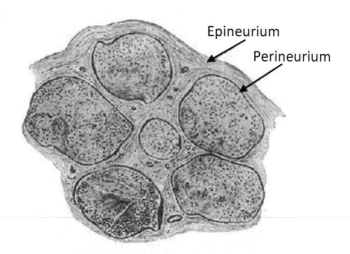

Epineurium
Perineurium

Gray's Anatomy - Originally published in 1918

Mostly it encloses structures to support them and to segregate them from other structures, but it can also serve to allow sliding of one structure beside another. Problems arise when fascia becomes shortened, or when the fascia of one structure becomes glued to the fascia of another structure. For example, after a Hysterectomy operation most people are familiar with the development of adhesions which form when white blood cells respond to the presence of residual blood and try and "heal" the injury by gluing everything together in the vicinity. When the Intestinal Tract becomes glued to itself or to the Abdominal Wall this restricts normal movement stimulating pain fibers and causing pain. What is not so obvious is that analogous problems are forming throughout the body even without an operation as a precipitating event. We see the same thing with Endometriosis which causes inflammation and bleeding inside the Abdominal Cavity. Another common source of abnormal fascia is trauma. We mentioned operations, which are an iatrogenic source of adhesions, but any bruising can produce a similar result.

It appears as though the Fibroblasts (cells that make connective tissue) are always gluing everything in the body. The reason that we have not been completely cocooned in Fascia is that when we move we tear it up. Thus Fascia is only left more permanently at the limits of our range of motion forming a support structure in those areas. However, as we become more and more sedentary we slowly become enclosed in its web and our motions become increasingly restricted. Motion that was once restricted by choice becomes structurally fixed. This is most markedly illustrated when a cast is put on a limb. If the cast is left on too long the limb will become Fibrotic and immobile. I once had a patient that came to me because her doctor had put her leg in a cast for six months. When it was taken off she could not move her foot and was unable to walk. Through persistence she was able to move slowly and carefully, but could no longer run or go long distances. I worked with her for months, before we could restore some semblance of normal function.

It is not just blood oxygenation that stimulates fibroblasts. It appears that inflammation also stimulates them to action. A related issue is that inflammation usually leads to immobility, which amplifies its effect. But inflammation alone seems to be enough. One of the commonest sources of abnormal fascia comes from tight muscles and their relationship to nerves. Nerves should slide easily through muscle tissue. When the muscles are relaxed it minimizes friction as there are no hard surfaces to rub against. However, when muscles are chronically tight the sliding of nerves under the muscle results in excess rubbing. We can hypothesize a low grade inflammation resulting from this friction, which is interpreted as an injury by the fibroblasts. They respond to this by forming fibrous adhesions between the nerve and the associated muscle fascia. Now when movement occurs the nerve no longer slides freely under the muscle, but is held in place by the adhesions. Tying the nerve and muscle together in an abnormal relationship is an irritant to the nerve, causing common symptoms such as Carpal Tunnel and Restless Leg Syndrome, in addition to others.

The first individual to fully comprehend the significance of Fascia in health was Dr. Ida Rolf. Although trained as a chemist, in the 1930s she began applying her scientific training to health problems by working on individuals who had trouble getting into various Yoga postures. Through exposure to Osteopathic and Chiropractic Medicine and other forms of natural healing she developed the ideas and techniques that have become known as Rolfing Structural Integration. In short, she realized that Fascia could become dysfunctional and restrict motion and posture causing pain and even disease. Her technique consisted of ten one-hour sessions in which the practitioner systematically addresses the restrictions throughout the body. The effects on posture and freedom of motion can be striking.

Her ideas were refined beyond addressing postural issues by Dr. Michael Leahy, a Chiropractor. He has patented his technique as Active Release Technique or ART. While Dr. Rolf's ideas are well suited to correcting issues with general posture, Dr. Leahy has refined specific solutions to such problems such as shoulder pain, Carpal Tunnel, various Tendonitises and athletic issues. Trained as an Aeronautical Engineer his techniques exhibit extreme precision which will be hard to improve. The problem that ART Practitioners encounter is diagnostic, finding the exact location of adhesions. Without precision in this area, large areas of the nerve-muscle interface must be treated. This problem has been solved with the application of Applied Kinesiology Muscle Testing to ART, the system developed by Dr. George Goodheart. It turns out that nerve adhesions disturb the electromagnetic field of the nerve to which large muscles are sensitive. They respond in the same way as other forms of therapy localization. A doctor skilled in AK can easily locate the exact location of adhesions and resolve them promptly with ART. Together they form the best MyoFascial Technology available.

Abdominal Health

It has been said repeatedly that death begins in the colon. In our culture, most men and women develop a pot belly in their later 40s or early 50s that stays with them for the rest of their life. Nobody feels good with a belly swollen with fat and fecal matter. Why does this happen?

For most of this we need to look no farther than the American Lifestyle and fast food diet that has become a plague on our culture. This diet is characterized by a lack of nutrients, high fat and sugar, and a lack of fiber. The last of these, lack of fiber, we will take up first. There are two kinds of fiber, soluble and insoluble, and they play different roles in the intestinal tract. Soluble fiber's main function is to hold water in the Intestinal Tract. If you eat a bowl of corn meal mush, you add a little corn meal to a lot of water to get a lot of mush. This forms a water-binding medium that softens the stool and allows fluid movement and absorption of toxins that need to be excreted.

Anyone with hard stools is low on soluble fiber. Without soluble fiber we become constipated. Insoluble fiber has a totally different function. It mainly serves to bind the stool into a solid mass that can be pushed through the intestinal lumen by peristalsis.

Without insoluble fiber the stool becomes either watery without structure, or divided into hard lumps as occurs with the digestion of meat without fiber. Insoluble fiber is what creates a short transit time. You can test this by eating a beet and waiting for a red stool to exit the other end. If it takes more than 24 hours then you are constipated and need more insoluble fiber.

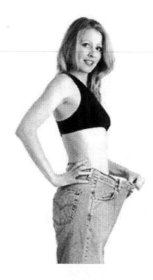

Insoluble fiber comes naturally in the form of salad and raw vegetables. This is really the only form of insoluble fiber that actually works. There are many commercial products of insoluble fiber composed primarily of ground psyllium husks. In my opinion this is a bad idea because the structural benefits of salad are completely lost and the stool exits the far end as a semi-liquid toothpaste. This may shorten transit time over no fiber at all, but is grossly inferior to a green salad. Inside the intestine, it is dysfunctional as the stool has no integrity and will bulge when pushed against with peristaltic action. This bulging action will cause the Intestinal Tract to expand Lumen size by stretching the connective tissue and smooth muscle of the intestinal wall.

This pushing against the intestinal wall when combined with infection can lead to serious health problems. The reason for this is several infectious agents eat connective tissue and will weaken the structural integrity of the intestinal wall.

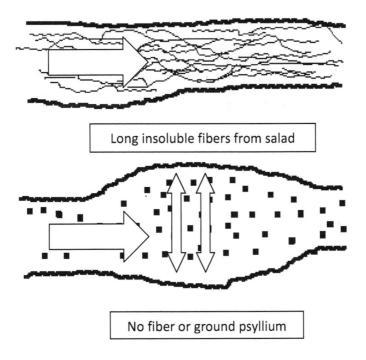

Long insoluble fibers from salad

No fiber or ground psyllium

Infections that like to eat connective tissue include Fungal, Mycoplasmic and Trematode infestations. Some bacteria also secrete Proteolytic enzymes that can degrade connective tissue. Once the Lumen wall is weakened it will bulge outward forming what are known as Diverticuli. On a barium X-Ray they appear as small hollow mushrooms. Because the normal flow of the intestinal matter bypasses the Diverticuli they tend to become infected with any microbes that occupy them first. Infection is a bridge to far more serious disease manifestation.

Many Holistic Practitioners have adopted the model of intestinal degeneration that describes this deterioration as due to an accumulated coating of the interior Lumen with impacted matter.

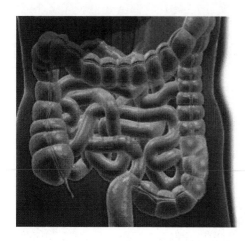

Diverticula

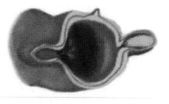

Blood   Diverticulitis

According to this view the coating develops from years of poor eating and abuse. As it forms, it blocks absorption of nutrients and becomes saturated with toxins and infection leading to poor health. I have talked to several Gastroenterologists who have done many thousands of endoscopic exams of the colon and they tell me that they have never seen any impactions like this. I believe this idea originated with Dr. Bernard Jensen, of Iridology fame, who published a book on colon cleansing showing pictures of long tubes of dark matter excreted from the intestine during colonic cleansing. Apparently, what is happening in these cases that he documented, is an artifact of the cleansing process that he recommends. As part of his cleansing program he encourages consuming clay along with green powders. This apparently bonds with the mucus on the Intestinal Lining forming this impacted material. It does not exist, to my knowledge, among people who do not consume clay.

Therefore, it should not be the goal of intestinal cleansing to rid ourselves of this fictitious coating. It should be to keep the cells of the Lumen healthy so Diverticuli do not form, and so the intestine can function properly by absorbing the nutrients we need and by forming an effective barrier against things we do not need. If Diverticuli already exist, then they need to be kept free of infection with fiber and healthy intestinal flora.

Obesity

Symptoms associated with Obesity such as High Cholesterol, High Triglycerides, Heart Disease, Stroke and Type II Diabetes are all part of what is called Syndrome X. These are all symptoms of Insulin Resistance, meaning that the Insulin receptors throughout the body are increasingly unresponsive to Insulin, the hormone that drives blood sugar into the cells for use. Factors that are known to influence this expression of physiological decline include depressed nutritional intake, high intake of fats and refined carbohydrates, and lack of exercise. The dominant theory to account for this problem is an overexposure to refined carbohydrates that keep blood sugar and insulin high, thus dulling the insulin receptors. More recently a new theory has emerged for reversing Diabetes, published in a book by Dr. Neal Barnard, the theory presents the idea that Insulin Resistance is actually due to a congestion of Insulin Receptors by saturated fat, not carbohydrates. Once clogged, the receptors no longer respond to Insulin and cause the observed rise in blood sugar. According to Dr. Barnard studies done to test the validity of this idea placed patients on diets that either restricted carbohydrates, or restricted fats. The low fat diets always win.

What does exercise have to offer overweight individuals? First, there are two types of exercise that are of value. The first is exercise that involves some bouncing activity such as running or working out on a trampoline or even a hula hoop. Anything that jiggles the intestinal tract will stimulate the stretch receptors in the intestinal wall causing the smooth muscle to contract. This increases peristalsis as well as narrowing the Intestinal Lumen if it has become enlarged. It will tone the intestine and shorten transit time.

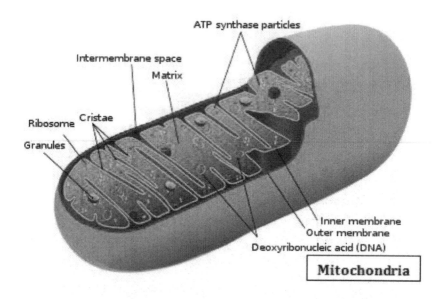

Mitochondria

Usually bouncing exercises are aerobic. This aerobic feature will increase the production of one key molecule called IGC-Alpha 1. This molecule is a key player in increasing the number of Mitochondria in your body. Resistance exercise apparently does not do this as much. Mitochondria are the energy producing organelles of your cells that excrete another molecule called ATP. ATP functions like a molecular battery holding the electrons that are used to run all functions of your body.

The second type of exercise that is of value is weight resistance exercise. This builds muscle mass which burns fat, keeping you fit.

Weight resistance exercise also stimulates the production of new Insulin Receptors, thus providing a direct avenue to reducing Insulin Resistance. As mentioned earlier, if the weight exercise is done with great intensity it stimulates the release of hormones beneficial to health. These include Growth Hormone and Testosterone.

Glycation

Most people notice that their eyesight becomes progressively weaker as they age. This is because the lens in their eyes is slowly becoming stiffer and will no longer stretch when pulled on by the muscles surrounding it that allow for visual accommodation. What most people don't know is that their heart is going through the same process. What happens is that both the eye and heart are being Glycated. It turns out that sugar and protein bond with each other and cause a stiffening of the tissues involved. This process does not just occur in these two organs, but occurs throughout the body to a lesser degree. Stopping this process is one of the unsolved problems in preventing aging. The only substance I am aware of that impacts this is an Amino Acid called Carnosine. When you are young your body has lots of it, but as you age the levels slowly decline. It is expensive, but it can be purchased and taken orally. Until something better comes along, I would recommend taking it as a supplement and extending longevity for your heart and eyes.

On Comfort Foods and Uncomfortable Meditations

The fact that people will take things into their bodies that are knowingly harmful to them is both practically and philosophically perplexing. Why would a being exist who knowingly consumes foods that are self-destructive? What does this self-destructive impulse consist of? To answer this we need to consider this from two perspectives; how this condition evolved in the first place, and why it is not resolved once created.

If we take a specific example of this, say eating a plate of French Fries, we would probably all agree that we eat it because it tastes good and is satisfying. However, this is a superficial explanation as it does not consider why we have evolved to enjoy something devoid of meaningful nutrition. Choices like this would eventually weaken our survival capacity.

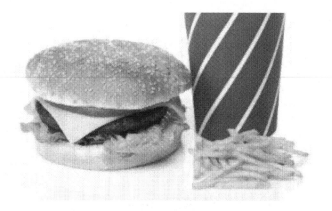

Dr. Francis Pottenger, M.D. did studies on cats between 1932 and 1942 that provides an analogy to our situation. He fed two groups of cats an identical diet which consisted largely of meat, except that for one group the meat was cooked. The cooking destroys the protein and makes it unusable by the body. This creates a type of nutritionally-depleted food. He then followed them for several generations and noted changes in their health. The cooked meat cats first developed Arthritis, then loss of coordination, then Epilepsy, and then genetic defects such as an extra toe. The raw meat cats all remained healthy. This is only one example of nutritional depletion, but we are fools if we don't learn from it. In most cases, eating raw food (uncooked foods) is the healthiest way to eat as we have not adapted physiologically to the changed chemistry of cooking. We cook to kill parasites, preserve foods and sometimes to release nutrients from their cellulose encasements in plant fiber, but we should always eat a good part of our diet raw.

We have to start looking at this by confronting the fact that taste is a poor guide for nutrition. In fact, the entire fast food industry has hired an army of PhDs to study taste in order to capitalize on this perceptual failure, and we can see the consequences of this manipulation in the overweight and sick population that limps through life full of soft drinks, fatty foods and empty calories. But regardless, of who is trying to manipulate us for profit, we are caught in a battle between what our tastes tell us to do and what we need to do to build health. Why would taste evolve to betray our health? If we entered a wilderness area and found the population of animals overweight, Arthritic, riddled with cardiovascular problems and one-third dying of Cancer, we would immediately think there is something wrong with the environment. But we choose instead to look for a "cure" for these diseases, as though these problems did not have a context. The drug industry asks the question, "What drug would keep us healthy while we live off soft drinks and junk food?" I can see where this would take countless billions of dollars to solve scientifically, if it can be done at all. The health food industry has taken a different approach and asks a different question, "What food and lifestyle choices are we making to create these problems?" This does not take much money to fix.

There are instances where taste seems to work properly. For example, if I am extremely hungry I will tend to imagine foods that would satisfy me. I do not dream of a Hot Fudge Sundae. This tells us that there is a meaningful channel between taste and real need, but it often fails. Simple reasoning tells us why this channel is not working for us anymore.

Most of our genetic adaptations occurred over long time periods and for most of our ancestral existence we lived in an environment where we were tuned more closely to our environment. Think of a deer in a forest, most everything he chooses to eat is healthy. There are no French Fries or Cokes. The environment contains only young green shoots and clean water. Our ancestors used to live off the same things. But now our environment has been transformed by culture and technology, and it has changed much faster than we can possibly evolve physiologically. In a sense, our illnesses are a form of culture shock. We have not learned to adapt to the world we have created or sense its danger, so we act like fools.

But this insight does not tell us why we do not respond to the knowledge we have of the foods we are eating. In fact, people that stop the intake of these foods often find they are confronted by tensions and anxiety. Food has a calming effect allowing us to work and sleep with more ease. We understand that food stimulates the Parasympathetic system to promote digestion, and the Parasympathetic system is relaxing. But this is the consequence of eating anything and does not explain choosing fast foods.

These foods are heavily promoted by our culture by advertising and by their ubiquitous presence. Most aspects of culture are actively maintained by constant reinforcement. Internally, we constantly talk to ourselves and externally we are reinforced constantly by similar bombardment of cultural reminders. This suggests an obvious strategy to combat this programming, by choosing to expose ourselves to programming we ourselves have chosen through reading and education. This does work, however, there is another strategy that is more profound and necessary for us to mature as individuals to develop a presence in ourselves that reaches outside the habitual culture we are imbedded in. It is common knowledge that people who find themselves adrift alone in a raft following a maritime accident often start hallucinating. Dr. Timothy Leary has commented that this is due to symbol deprivation, meaning that if the brain is starved of cultural references it starts to function outside our habitual norms and new forms of experience emerge. Although some cultures have established ritual activities to seek these experiences, such as vision quests or meditation, to most people this is a threatening and uncomfortable experience. We can experience great anxiety as we move from the habitual culturally bound existence to the free emergence of perceptual gestalts in spontaneous awareness.

One thing we can easily notice about ourselves is that we are rarely still. Our minds are filled with stories we tell ourselves and activities that fill our time. If we try and turn it all off we find it difficult to do. The truth is that there is a compulsory nature to these self preoccupying activities. They can only be stopped with persistent effort, such as occurs in meditation, something most of us have never truly made the effort to do. So what is this boundary into stillness about? Why can't we just decide to enjoy stillness and be in it? If we cross the boundary and force ourselves to be still we feel the pressure to turn back. We twitch and become uncomfortable and our mind starts talking and daydreaming. What is this all about?

If we move away from the example of meditation and search for other instances when we feel anxious we notice they occur when we are dealing with the unexpected, where we don't know what the outcome will be, and there is something at stake. But how would this apply if we are simply sitting alone just trying to be still? What could be at stake, and what outcome are we uncertain about?

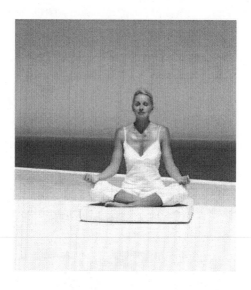

To answer that let's start with the concepts of fantasy and internal dialogue. If we observe them we will notice that they largely deal with daily life and the culture around us. For example, I might think "What will I say? What will happen?". Perhaps we might rehearse a conversation we would like to have with someone to whom we are attracted. These are obviously efforts to rehearse for life so we will be better prepared. So this makes a little more sense because we are abandoning our preparation for daily life. So we are afraid of experiencing life without having a prepared routine. It is stage fright, in a Shakespearean sense, "Life is a Stage".

To take another example, if we are approaching someone that we are attracted to, what are we nervous about? Obviously, failure and the way that feels, but what happens when we feel that way? We are afraid it will take the wind out of us and reduce our capacity to reach out, thus reducing our survival ability. Is something like this happening when we are sitting alone? Since in meditation when we are dealing primarily with perception we might ask ourselves what we might perceive that would deflate us and weaken our power.

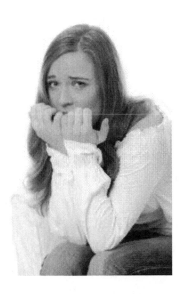

To understand what is lost try and talk to someone about your experiences that occur in meditation, especially someone who does not involve themselves in these activities. It takes some effort to formulate what you are going to say and then you might not be understood. You certainly run the risk of being thought of as "weird". In a way, you need to develop a new form of contact with the person you are trying to talk to, unless they already had the experience you are referring to. You need to feel your way together again.

Junk food, because of its commonality, because of its habitual and familiar nature, serves as a communion with our culture and all the social bonds associated with it. Our mind habitually moves towards it. We use foods like this all the time; at Thanksgiving to form communion with our family, at weddings, at business meetings and even Catholic Communion to have connection with Christ. With each sensuous bite we rejoin our group and reinforce the world our social bonds use for currency. When we travel to foreign lands, like China, and we see a McDonald's, why do we choose to eat there? This is probably the worst food in China, yet many of us are happy to participate in this ritual. Eating something familiar has a sweet comforting quality about it. It makes us feel at home. Much junk food is laced with sugar and this awakens the links of sweetness to love.

There are synthetic connections between sweetness and love and we often call our lover Honey or Sweetheart, and this is why we eat sweets to comfort ourselves. We even call these foods "comfort foods." It creates a hypnosis that the fast food industry has built up carefully to keep you buying and consuming these foods.

But what is the positive side of stepping outside this habitual world? Years ago, I watched an interesting video of a young black Leopard that had just separated from his mother and was for the first time on his own in the jungle. He is hungry to the point of starvation, and one of the first things he runs across is a large King Cobra. The young cat approaches the snake thinking he would make a great meal. Then he stops for several long minutes. The snake, reared up with its hood spread, and the hungry cat poised motionless stare at each other across an electric space. Suddenly the tension is broken and the cat turns around and walks away. How did he know he was facing death, having never seen a Cobra before? How did he know about the poison?

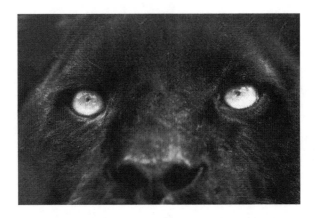

However he did it, it was done with careful meditation and stillness and he learned something completely new. This ability is something we all have to some degree. I believe we can do what that young black Panther did with anything we are approaching, if we see directly without social conditioning, but obviously this does not usually happen.

What can we learn from this? First, these experiences take you out of the social norm and your cultural comforts. You end up standing by yourself and living with your raw experience, not knowing how it will reintegrate with your social world. But on the other side of the fence there may be something positive about what you see. Perhaps for a moment, you look at the world like that young leopard and perceive something that reveals a bit of truth directly. Perhaps you see what junk food really is. Perhaps you are inspired on how to communicate in a relationship. Perhaps you realize what you could become. These experiences allow us to revision our purpose and envelope our activities in meaning.

So getting back to the original question about why taste deceives you about choosing foods, we can better sense why we might enjoy empty nutrient foods even though they are not great for us. It is like participating in a social catharsis of taste. If we look at the psychology behind decisions that lead to symptoms, we will often find anxieties of this nature, anxieties related to separation from our social matrix. It is the compost that fuels our addictions and keeps us in our habitual culture, and so doing preserves the comfort of our social bonds. Very often also there are early experiences of social loss and we unconsciously seek to avoid restimulation and reliving those experiences, so we eat our comfort foods.

The reason why people get into health foods and supplements is that they have developed their vision of what is possible by living this way rather than following the habit patterns formed by the fast food industry. In a sense, they are forming a new culture of their own making. They have taken the reins of their lives and direct it based on their own instincts. Sometimes this happens after a major illness, especially if correct eating has been a factor in recovery. But anyone can do this. I often tell patients that it is more useful to imagine how a food will feel in your body after it is eaten, rather than thinking about how it will taste before we eat it.

Nutrition and Telomeres

We tend to have the view that genetics are fixed unalterable influences on our health and nutrition works around these genetic determinants. This is a half truth. The genetic make-up is referred to as our genotype. The expression of this genetic make-up is referred to as the Phenotype. So, for example, two people with identical genes may look very different according to their lifestyle, one may be fat and the other skinny.

In addition, to the expression as Phenotypes, there is also evidence that the genes themselves can be influenced by environmental influences, including supplementation. This can take several forms which might include repair of DNA, or protection of DNA from damage, or rebuilding and lengthening Telomeres. A Telomere is the end chain on DNA which shortens each time an individual cell divides. When the Telomere is gone cell division stops and the cell becomes old. There was a recent study published in the American Journal of Clinical Nutrition that found individuals who take multivitamins had an average Telomere length 5.1% longer than those that do not take multivitamins.

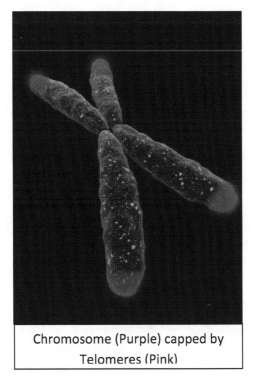

Chromosome (Purple) capped by
Telomeres (Pink)

This raises the question that if multivitamins preserve Telomeres, perhaps nutrition could be refined to produce a larger effect? What about the detrimental effects of nutrients that reduce the length of Telomeres? There is evidence that aspects of diet can shorten Telomeres. For example, it has been demonstrated that a diet that includes processed meats, such as salami and hot dogs, will result in shorter Telomeres. This study published in The American Journal of Clinical Nutrition did not find any other correlations between diet and Telomeres, but this is almost certainly not the case.

For example, another article published in the Journal of Pathology found shortened Telomeres in the Esophagus of drinkers, so we can assume this is due to alcohol Free Radical damage.

Reviewing the research has made it obvious that Telomere length is influenced by a wide variety of lifestyle factors including hormones, diet, stress, infection, disease, meditation and exercise. However, one concept stands out to integrate these various elements; the idea of oxidative stress. In fact, Telomere length has been suggested as a marker for Oxidative Stress.

What is Oxidative Stress? This is the body's lack of ability to deal with reactive oxygen radicals produced through normal metabolic functioning or through other physiological stressors.

This means that various aspects of metabolism produce Free Radicals which tear the body down. The factors that produce Free Radicals are on one side of the equation and factors that rebuild the body are on the other. The greater the general efficiency of the body the less damage produced by this process. Oxidative Stress will also attack the DNA and its Telomeres.

Short Telomeres are prognostic for disease risk in Cancer as well as progression and mortality of the disease. Short Telomeres are also reflected in Cardiac Disease, Atherosclerosis, Insulin Deficient Diabetes, Cataracts, Muscle Loss, Ulcerative Colitis, Rheumatoid Arthritis, Obesity, increases in Homocystine and senescence of the immune system. It has been found that individuals with Rheumatoid Arthritis have an immune system 20 years older than individuals without the disease.

However, Telomeres can be lengthened, not just preserved. Individuals with Prostate Cancer who underwent significant lifestyle changes experienced lengthening of Telomeres along with decreases in LD Lipoprotein and Cholesterol, and other stress indicators. It has been found that women have longer Telomeres than men. This could be due to higher levels of Estrogen which is known to lengthen Telomeres. There are a number of other hormones and supplements that positively influence Telomerase, the enzyme that increases Telomeres. These include Niacin, Carnosine, NAC (N-Acetyl Cysteine) and Tocotrienols. There are undoubtedly many more. One supplement that may have a dramatic impact on Telomeres is Co-Enzyme Q-10. Life Extension published research on this enzyme revealing that it extended youth in young mice by 45% when they were given it from infancy. This may well occur by lengthening the Telomeres. We will wait for further research. Meanwhile, this is a supplement everyone should be taking.

If you are thinking of taking it you should know there are two types; Ubiquinone and Ubiquinol. The latter is the better one and is 8 times better absorbed.

The issue of Telomeres brings up the question of how much life can be extended by lifestyle changes. I have been observing my patients for many years and I have the general impression that someone with a lifestyle slanted towards healthy habits can add 20 years of youth. In the end, I am most interested and concerned with "healthspan" or "youthspan" more than lifespan, but the two likely have some relationship. I do not imagine too many people with long unhealthy lives. I am sure 20 years is not the upper limit for youth expansion as there is always new information developing on how better to live and eat. Because genetic research is evolving so fast it is wise to be as healthy as possible to increase the possibility of a long life. Who knows what the upper limit will be? If Co-Q 10 can add nearly 50 per cent to youth, perhaps even that could be greatly extended if a total lifestyle upgrade was instituted. This would allow us to live long enough to take advantage of the new advances in science.

Longevity Intelligence

All of the available information on health and longevity as well as emerging scientific breakthroughs will be of no use unless the wisdom and intelligence is developed to recognize and to make use of it. Thus arises the need to cultivate a mindset to allow absorption of the right kind of knowledge, and consequently the right motivation to develop it. Some of this is common sense, but it is impossible to know what to do without information, so the most obvious thing is to keep absorbing information that will help you. I recommend keeping a health book near you to read little bits whenever a free moment arises. It will keep you informed and interested.

However, an equally important faculty to develop is a sense of what your body needs. Some people are born with this already quite developed. For example, I often see teenage girls working in health food stores and restaurants. With little formal education they seem to instinctively gravitate towards what is healthy. Many formally trained doctors have little of this sense. This is an instinct that can be developed through self observation and education.

You can sense when you need digestive enzymes, Vitamin C or Probiotics. Often this occurs when you feel a stress in your body and learn what cures it by experimentation. Sometimes someone will teach you something helpful and you will remember it. These experiences will accumulate and fuse into a wisdom about health. This is essential if you wish a long healthspan.

Toxicity and Detoxification

We live in an increasingly polluted world. According to the World Health Organization Cancer rates worldwide are expected to increase 50 per cent by 2020. This used to be a rare disease. All around the world male fertility is in sharp decline. According to an Italian study done at the University of Pizza Italian men have 50 per cent fewer active sperm than they did in the 1970s. The Swedish doctor Niels Skakkebaek has stated that global male sperm count has decreased one per cent per year since the 1930s. Amphibians such as frogs are disappearing around the world. According to the Alzheimer's Association rates for Alzheimer's Disease have increased 46.1 per cent between 2000 and 2006. It is a little scary if you are aware of these things and care about future generations.

Unfortunately, most of these toxins can neither be seen nor felt. They exist as an invisible danger, both to yourself and to your loved ones. Some of these toxins are dumped into our diet on purpose through the efforts of misguided public officials. An example of this is Fluoride which is put into our drinking water.

Fluoride is known to cause Cancer and loss of IQ in children. To learn more, please review my article at NaturalCureDoctor.com. Others are added into foods for practical reasons, although short sighted.   An example of this is insecticides sprayed on our vegetables.   Scientific American published an article a few years back estimating that half of all Cancers are caused by these chemicals in our food.

Yet, we spend billions looking for a "cause" of Cancer without addressing the fact that we are the "cause."   We should all be supporting organic farming and any efforts to clean the environment.   Another problem is the use of antibiotics in the cattle and chicken industry.

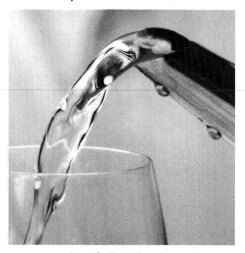

Image by Jenny Downing

This overuse promotes the evolution of antibiotic resistant strains of bacteria that we can no longer control with our medicines. We also have problems with heavy metals, particularly Mercury which has contaminated all of our oceans and has made fish, one of our most important sources of food, dangerous to eat. The list goes on and on. There does not seem to be the political will to correct these problems, most likely because of the political influence of corporations that are benefiting financially from this pollution. How short-sighted are we? We allow ourselves to be manipulated so a few people can make a lot of money.

Anyone who does not make an effort to eat organic vegetables and meats is needlessly putting themselves at risk. You cannot eliminate all toxins doing this, but it surely is a big help. Secondly, we need to drink water that has been purified by distillation and filtration. According to Dr. Colgan of the Colgan Institute there are 2,500 contaminants in drinking water and the FDA only monitors a few. He maintains that competitors in the Olympic Games cannot win if they drink tap water due to the contaminants. Thirdly, we need to avoid plastic drinking containers and heating foods and liquids in plastic containers. All plastics leak chemicals that are Estrogen mimics. And fourth, we need to avoid exposure to toxic household sprays and cleaning materials. These steps are all essential.

We know the toxicity exists, but what should we do to eliminate what has already entered our body? Detoxification in the body occurs in two Phases. In Phase 1, the toxins are oxidized by P450 enzymes, often making the products of this reaction more toxic than the original toxins. However, this stage is essential to detoxify the body. Both Phase 1 and 2 can be tested to determine which pathways are disturbed. Phase 1 detoxification can be up-regulated by drinking coffee, if it is under functioning. Dr. Jeffrey Bland of Metagenics fame has indicated that this may be the mechanism by which coffee is protective against pathologies like Parkinson's disease. If Phase 2 is under functioning and Phase 1 is working well a condition can be created called pathological detoxification in which these harmful products of Phase 1 accumulate. Phase 2 involves several types of reactions which make the toxins water soluble so they can be excreted from the body, especially through the kidneys. Glutathione is the only enzyme that functions in both Phase 1 and Phase 2, so you can never go wrong raising its levels in the body. There are a number of nutrients that raise Glutathione, but the main one is the Amino Acid L-Cystine.

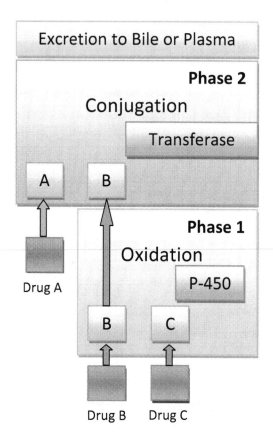

Other nutrients that likely have a positive effect include the antioxidant Alpha Lipoic Acid, the herb Milk Thistle or its extract Silymarin, and the insect eating mushroom Cordycepts.

This is a good combination to be taken on a daily basis to keep detoxification through Glutathione functioning at a high level. Detoxification of heavy metals involves a somewhat different strategy. Sulfur containing compounds like DMSA are effective as chelating agents, but the metals are very prone to being reabsorbed from the intestinal tract unless steps are taken to block this auto-contamination.

When detoxifying heavy metals we usually increase the consumption of fiber as well as taking green clay on a cyclical basis. This strategy will result in a rapid drop of heavy metals when retested. Other factors that help detoxification are exercise and sweating, or long infrared sauna especially if combined with exercise. The effect of this combination can be wonderful and renewing.

You can feel reborn energetically after a good detox. Sometimes this can be amplified by using Niacin at doses that cause vasodialation. Other helpful aids can be colonics and ionic foot baths. Sometimes taking bile can help stimulate the flow of bile through the liver picking up toxins on the way. As mentioned, the bile must be bound by fiber in the intestinal tract to prevent re-absorption.

Detoxifying can be both preventative and curative for a vast array of problems. With the help of a medical professional this can be an avenue for treating Cancer, as is done at the Gerson Institute. For the rest of us it can rid us of pains and revive our sagging energy.

Chronic Inflammation

One of the most insidious processes leading to pain and aging is Chronic Inflammation. There are multiple possible causes, but the ones most commonly recognized are infections, toxins, acidic diet and stress. Chronic Inflammation is like stress in that multiple lesser causes are cumulative. Some diseases, like Fibromyalgia usually have multiple factors involved, all of which need to be corrected in order to realize a resolution of the problem. Chronic Inflammation is itself a stressor and can be a significant factor leading to Immune and Adrenal exhaustion, thus further aggravating the inflammatory state. It will interact with almost any other problem that is manifesting in the body to make it worse. Chronic Inflammation is associated with multiple diseases, including Cancer, Arthritis, Osteoporosis, Alzheimer's Disease and Cardiovascular Disease, which are the worst scourges of mankind. It is imperative to find and treat its causes to cool its fires. A general marker of Chronic Inflammation is C-Reactive Protein which can easily be tested for. But usually patients who are suffering from Chronic Inflammation will have many signs of its presence including body and muscle soreness, sore joints, fatigue and cardiovascular distress.

The factors that cause inflammation such as infection, Autoimmune Diseases and toxins, have been briefly addressed earlier, but acidic diet and Adrenal exhaustion have not. The acidity of the body is buffered by the chemistry of the blood to keep it within a normal range. Having said that, schools of Natural Healing have always maintained that this buffering system is preserved at the expense of your bones, which lose Calcium, and at the expense of other minerals in the body. Primarily the body is alkalinized by minerals from vegetables and supplements, and by reducing consumption of foods that have an acid ash. By acid ash we do not mean whether the food itself is acidic, like grapefruit juice, but whether the ash of the food, after it has been metabolized, is acidic. The main foods that produce an acid ash are grains and protein. It is believed that limiting these foods will help soothe an acidic body.

The other factor of the Adrenal Glands is important for controlling inflammation as they produce Cortisol which has strong anti-inflammatory effects. Because the Adrenals produce Cortisol in response to stress, including physiological stressors, it can eventually exhaust its capacity to make this hormone if the stressor is too persistent. Once this happens, the body will have many signs of this exhaustion, but among them is a lack of capacity to deal with inflammation.

If the Adrenals are functioning normally, they produce the bulk of their Cortisol first thing in the morning in a large flush. So Cortisol should be high in the morning and slowly decline as the day progresses, until evening when it is very low. This cycle is important as Cortisol raises blood glucose. If it is high in the evening, then it will interfere with sleep as higher blood sugar is activating to the nervous system and will make sleep difficult. If an individual cannot sleep it will produce more stress, further exhausting the Adrenals and reducing the body's capacity to deal with inflammation. Therefore, in dealing with the Adrenals, both the chronic stressors, as well as the cycle of hormone release, need to be resolved.

Pain Is Not Always What It Seems

As I have presented in the case histories the problem of pain is better understood and recognized as being linked to many hidden stresses in the body, so pain is often not conceived causally as a local event. For patients who have problems that do not seem to resolve themselves by simple exercise, physical therapy, or adjusting techniques, I hope these case histories will help them find a real resolution. Many of the insights presented here have been the direct result of Dr. Goodheart's wonderful discoveries about the potential of Muscle Testing and its capacity to connect seemingly unrelated events in the body.

I have presented anti-aging as a philosophy to reduce the potential of disease and pain. This is a field worth keeping your pulse tuned into, as it will soon be changing the world and your own prospects for extended youth.

Testimonials

I just finished reading your book. I thoroughly enjoyed it, and I found it filled with loads of insightful information. I think that the explanation of how dysfunction is related to pain and then to disease is very important to health care in general. Things such as stress, persistent inflammation, symbol deprivation and diet have been neatly tied together in your book. I tend to think that this book needs to be read and re-read for better digestion. It can also serve as a reference manual for people to better self diagnose the Secret of their own Pain. P.S. thank you again for your passion for healing, and for all the wonderful insights.

~Kirk~

****

At age 92, I credit much of my good health to my chief health consultant, Dr. Robert Janda. He uses a number of effective techniques to discover and treat various physical problems, and he has also sent me to other excellent doctors from time to time. He has my deep appreciation and I am pleased to recommend him.

Pierce C. Ommanney, PhD

****

Through the way you have been treating me with patience, listened to my every complaint, and have been communicating, my body is healing from the inside out. Your determination and your compassion have given strength to my bones ......I thank you and appreciate you in every minute of my life.

Rona Ansary 2010

****

I continue to see Dr. Janda for various reasons, including nutritional advice. He is by far one of the most knowledgeable practitioners in his field. I learn so many things, simple things, to heal myself. I love Dr. Janda for helping me be healthy. And his bedside manner is exceptional. I have recommended him to many of my friends. He is all about helping people be the healthiest they can be. Thanks Dr. Janda!

Gwen Evans

****

Dr. Janda is the most sensitive Kinesiologist I have ever met. This gift gives him the ability to diagnose all kinds of problems quickly and accurately. Coupled with his extensive knowledge of how our bodies work and the roots of the pathologies we encounter, he has been able to help me through numerous difficulties, large and small, over the years. He's the number one defensive tool in my health kit!

Pat and Bob

****

I have been doing very well and my neck and back are, for the most part, pain free. But that is so far from where I was when I met Dr. Janda. Thank you seems inadequate. I met Dr. Janda in early 2003 after being diagnosed with Degenerative Disk Disease and was in chronic and severe pain. Doctors and Surgeons had told me that I would need to have my neck operated on and even then would still have pain and need medication for the rest of my life. Dr. Janda started treatment on my neck and he and his wonderful traction machine (my husband lovingly referred to as "the rack") did what doctors said couldn't be done. My neck is pain free and I am living a full and wonderful life pain and medication free! Thank you.

Lynne Oliveira PhD

****

I had a pain in my shoulder that prevented me from raising my right arm, to the point where I hardly moved it at all. Dr Janda, using his Rolfing Structural Integration method, completely healed that. I had had this pain for almost a year, and it has not returned after seven years.

Dave White, San Diego

****

I was fortunate enough to attend one of Dr. Janda's seminars years ago. Since then, I have consulted him regularly for various concerns that include infections and backaches. He has certainly helped to improve my physical health. And when necessary he has made excellent referrals to other doctors. I highly recommend him to all for preventative care, acute symptoms and chronic problems.

M. Mycena, PhD

****

Dr Janda is a walking encyclopedia and a perpetual student. When I met him he was a Chiropractor who was effective with Applied Kinesiology. His ongoing search for knowledge and his keeping up with new methods and advanced technology make him a very valuable health care provider.

Judith Epstein, Dr. Janda's Patient since 1992

****

I have played tennis for many years and was starting to suffer from tennis elbow. In the past this would have meant a long time of rest and no playing. I decided to see Dr. Janda about it, as he has helped me so many times with other issues in the past. In one session the pain was relieved, tennis elbow gone! I was back on the courts the next day!

John Valenzuela

****

I make my living as a faux and decorative painter. I was so worried one day when I had some strange nerve anomaly in my wrist, leaving my hand weakened. I didn't know if this would affect my ability to work.

The next day I saw Dr. Janda. I was a first time patient. I had a warm welcome and then he started evaluating and working on my hand. In all of five minutes my pain was gone and I was out the door. A little miracle. If you can call miracles little. Thank you Dr. Janda.

Kelley Havens

****

In my opinion, Dr. Janda is the very best in his field. I am constantly amazed at his ability to quickly zero-in on the specific problem area and administer the exact treatment needed. I am so grateful to have found such a wonderful and competent Applied Kinesiologist.

Karl Bergstrom

****

Dr. Janda displays a very non-conventional approach to the field of holistic medicine. I have gone to many holistic doctors in my life and have a very large field of comparison. Dr. Janda's level of presence as well as his awareness of his patients is very detailed and effective. His quality of listening, his awareness of symptoms and his ability to address these items is very rare. His diagnosis and treatment is so effective that at first it makes you skeptical that it could be true-- but then the results come quickly. Take, for example, my chronic bladder infections. I saw numerous medical doctors over a long period of time and could never really cure it. With Dr. Janda's treatment there was an immediate and abiding effect. It was really hard to believe and it was so freeing that it could be so simply treated. His power of knowledge, diagnosis and treatment is so effective that I bless him.

Rupa Ward, MFT

****

Dr. Janda, you are an inspiration! I am so truly grateful to you for all you're doing to help me heal once and for all! I can't express in words the gratitude I feel for you and your giving heart!

Dawn Depke

****

I have been going to Dr. Janda for over 10 years, when I feel any kind of pain on my side, neck, head, stomach, foot, hip, I mean everything! Dr. Janda finds the problem and gets me well right away. He is far beyond Chiropractic! He has so many skills and wisdom about health! One of his greatest skills is his expertise in Kinesiology. I can't say enough about Dr. Janda, my highest recommendations to anyone who wants quick holistic results!

Flory Park

****

Glossary

Achilles Tendonitis: This is inflammation of the Achilles Tendon that inserts into the heel.

Adrenal Glands: These are two small glands situated just above the kidneys that secrete several important hormones including Cortisol, sex hormones and Adrenaline.

Ah Shi Points: A term in Acupuncture Theory that refers to sore points on the body and are differentiated from established Acupuncture Points that have a predetermined location.

Allopathic Medicine: The dominant form of medicine practiced in the US and most industrial countries in the world.   It is based on concepts of attacking disease and is to be distinguished from Natural Medicine that promotes health to prevent disease.

Antibody: Also known as Immunoglobulins, a protein produced by plasma or B-cells, a type of white blood cell.   The antibody bonds with foreign microbes to neutralize them as part of the immune response.

Antioxidant: A class of molecules either produced within the body or eaten in foods that neutralizes free radicals. Free radicals are electron starved molecules that cause chemical damage in the body.

Applied Kinesiology: A school of Chiropractic developed by Dr. George Goodheart that uses Muscle Testing to elicit information about the health of the body.

Ascaris Lumbricoides: A type of microscopic round worm that is a parasite in the human body.

Association Points: A group of traditional acupuncture points present in two rows alongside the vertebrae on the back of the body. They reflect activities of organs.

Alarm Points: A group of traditional Acupuncture Points that appear on the front of the body, one for each organ. They tend to become sore with organ dysfunction.

Autoimmune Disease: A theory that some disease process are caused by the immune system attacking its own body.

Beauty: As used here it refers to the feeling of beauty that a person projects when the various systems of the body are healthy and in harmony.

"Bi-Digital O-Ring Testing": A system of hand Muscle Testing developed by Dr. Omura to determine health conditions in the body

C5: The fifth of seven vertebra in the neck

Carnosine: An Amino Acid found in the human body that has the property of blocking Glycation, the bonding of sugar to protein. It helps prevent stiffening of certain tissues such as the heart and cornea of the eye.

Carpal Tunnel: A tunnel of bones in the wrist that is known for trapping the median nerve causing a condition called Carpal Tunnel Syndrome. This causes pain, weakness and numbness in the hand. In fact, new research has shown this to be a mistaken concept and most "Carpal Tunnel" problems are caused elsewhere in the body.

Chlamydia trachomatis: A bacteria that infects the Urogenital system.

Chiropractic: A form of healing invented in the US by DD Palmer that promotes healing by treatment with the hands. At its origins the primary theory was to relieve nerve interference by adjusting the spine to correct Subluxations. Over the last 100 years it has incorporated other aspects of Natural Healing such as Nutrition and Herbology. It is currently the dominant form of Natural Healing in the US.

Chiropractic Manipulation: Also called Chiropractic Adjusting, involves correcting Subluxations through manual and mechanical force correctly applied to joints to reestablish their optimum mechanical function.

Chronic Fatigue: A diagnosis that refers to a condition of relentless long term fatigue, probably having multiple causes such as toxemia and infection.

Cortisol: A hormone produced by the Adrenal Gland that suppresses inflammation, raises blood sugar and helps the body adapt to stress, as well as other effects.

Costo-Sternal Pain: Pain in the joints on the chest where the ribs meet the sternum, the big flat bone in the center of the chest.

DHEA: A hormone produced by the Adrenal Glands that is the skeleton from which a cascade of other hormones such as Estrogen, Cortisol and Testosterone are made.

Dientemoeba Fragilis: A Protozoan parasite with a tail that infects the intestinal tract causing GI distress.

Dollard and Miller: Two psychologists who wrote a book that translates Psychoanalytic Theory into modern Learning Theory.

Dorsiflex: Flexion of the foot upward.

Dr. Yoshiaki Omura: An Oriental Medical Doctor given a US patent for "Bi-digital O-Ring Testing," a form of Muscle Testing used to determine health conditions in the body.

Estradiol: One of the three major Estrogens in the human body.

Extensor Muscles: Muscles that close the angle of a joint, as opposed to extensor muscles which open the joint.

Follicle Stimulating Hormone: A hormone produced by the Anterior Lobe of the Pituitary gland that stimulates the growth of the ovum-containing follicles in the ovary and activates sperm-forming cells —abbreviation **FSH**.

Frontal Bone: The bone in the skull that makes up the forehead.

Fasciculus Cuneatus and Graciis: Two nerve tracts in the spinal cord that carry proprioceptive information from the body to the brain.

Fascial Stretch: Fascia is connective tissue that occurs in sheets surrounding muscles and other tissues in the body. A fascial stretch is a manual technique that stretches the fascia.

Flexion Traction Table: A Chiropractic or osteopathic table that is used to stretch or traction the low back by using the table's ability to flex in the middle.

Foot Reflexologist: Someone who is trained to stimulate the reflex points on the bottom of the foot to facilitate healing.

Gamma Globulin Supplements: A supplement that contains Gamma Globulin, proteins that help the immune system fight infection.

Gastrocnemius Muscle: The muscle in the lower leg that forms the calf and allows you to stand on your toes.

Giardia: A Protozoa parasite that commonly infests the waterways in the US and causes severe intestinal distress.

Gliadin: A component of Gluten, a substance found in certain foods such as wheat. Some people have a genetic allergy to this substance which can cause brain damage and gastrointestinal problems.

Gluten: A protein found primarily in some grains that produces allergies in some people.

Glutathione: The main detoxifying agent and antioxidant found through out the body. High amounts are correlated with increased lifespan.

Glycation: The bonding of protein to sugar molecules producing "stiffness" of the tissues. This occurs naturally in the body and is responsible for loss of flexibility of the lens in the eye.

Hormone: A substance secreted by one organ in the body that targets another organ to stimulate some metabolic function.

Ileum Bone: Large bones in the pelvis that form the hips.

Inguinal Ligament: A ligament that runs across the front of the pelvis from the crest of the Ileum to the pubic symphysis. There is one ligament on each side and it forms part of the anatomy of the groin.

Kidney Yang: A concept in Chinese Medicine that refers to the active component of Kidney energy, not synonymous with the Kidney organ, and is described in modern terms as the activity of hormones secreted by the Adrenal Cortex.

Kidney Yin: A concept in Chinese Medicine that refers to the water filtering and detoxifying functions of the kidney.

L-Cystine: An Amino Acid that serves as a precursor to the formation of Glutathione.

Lovett Brother: A Chiropractic concept referring to a positional compensation between cervical and lumbar vertebrae so that if a lumbar vertebrae is malpositioned in one direction the corresponding cervical will rotate in the opposite direction.

LSA Testing: Short for "Limbic Stress Analysis", an electrical diagnostic technology used for screening problems in the body.

Lateral Spino-Thalamic Tract: A nerve tract in the spinal cord that carries pain information from the body to the brain.

Luteinizing Hormone: A hormone secreted by the Pituitary Gland in the brain that causes eggs to ripen in the ovary.

Lyme's Disease: A chronic disease caused by the bacteria Borrelia Burgdorferi and often transferred by the bite of a tic. Its symptoms are associated with Arthritis and Chronic Fatigue.

Melatonin: A hormone produced by the Pineal Gland at night that separates the metabolism of sleep from wakefulness. It has strong antioxidant properties protecting the DNA.

Meridian: A concept in Acupuncture describing the flow of energy in the body. There are 12 major Meridians, one for each organ of the body.

Micro Avulsion: A microscopic partial detachment of a tendon or ligament where it attaches to the bone.

Mitochondria: The organelle inside a cell that produces the energy for the cell and the body.

MRI: Stands for Magnetic Resonance Imaging which is a non-radiation form of imaging that can visualize the internal anatomy of the body in slices or planes.

Mycoplasm: A bacterial derived life form that has lost its cell wall and exists in the body as protoplasm only. They tend to be resistant to antibiotics and are difficult to visualize under a microscope. They may be responsible for diseases such as Rheumatoid Arthritis and Lyme's.

Myofascial: A term referring to muscles and their surrounding fascial sheets.

Musculoskeletal System: A term that includes the skeletal system and the muscular system.

Natural Healing: A school of healing that promotes the use of only natural techniques and substances such as herbs, manipulation and nutrition, as opposed to the use of drugs and surgery for healing. It is predominately espoused by Chiropractors, Naturopaths and Acupuncturists, but may be utilized by healers with any license.

Nerve Adhesions: Fibrous attachments that can develop between nerves and their surrounding tissue such that it restricts the natural sliding of the nerves during motion.

Nerve Brushing: A simple technique developed by Dr. Robert L. Janda to determine nerve irritation that involves brushing the skin over a nerve and using Applied Kinesiology Muscle Testing to test.

Nerve Entrapments: A general term used to describe any anatomical compression of a nerve that disturbs its function.

Neurotransmitters: Protein substances released from presynaptic nerve endings that cross the synaptic gap causing stimulation of the post synaptic nerve.

Nitric Oxide: A substance released by the intima of arteries that causes vasodilatation.

Orthopedic Testing: Traditional testing used by doctors to evaluate musculoskeletal problems.

Osteomylitis: Cancer of the bone.

Parasite: A foreign organism that lives on or inside the body often causing disease.

Parkinson's Disease: A disease produced by the destruction of the brain nuclei, the Substantia Niagra that causes symptoms of resting tremors and muscular rigidity.

Periostium: The fibrous sheath surrounding a bone.

Phylogenetic: The classification of organisms based on their evolutionary history.

Progestins: A manufactured artificial hormone like substance that mimics some of the properties of natural progesterone but unlike natural progesterone is carcinogenic.

Proprioception: The sensory ability to perceive position in space and motion.

Protozoa: A classification of single celled organisms bigger than bacteria and are represented by such creatures as amoeba and Giardia.

Pubic Symphesis: The joint where the two pubic bones join on the front of the body.

Pyriformis Muscle: A deep muscle in the buttocks that runs horizontally from the Sacrum to the Femur. It has special clinical significance as the Sciatic nerve runs through it or under it. Under some conditions it can trap or compress the nerve causing Sciatic Pain.

Pyriformis Syndrome: The clinical condition resulting from entrapment of the Sciatic Nerve under the Pyriformis Muscle.

Rectus Femoris: The large muscle on the front of the upper leg that flexes the leg or extends the knee.

Repetitive Strain Injury: A term used to describe inflammatory conditions caused by repeated motions each of which has little negative effect, but cumulatively can cause irritation.

Rotator Cuff: A ring of muscle attachments on the Upper Arm Bone (the Humerous) where it forms the shoulder joint.

Sacroiliac Joint: The joint between the Ilium Bone and the Sacrum in the posterior pelvis. It is prone to reflexive inflammation from intestinal infection.

Sciatica: Irritation of the Sciatic Nerve in the leg causing pain down the back of the leg.

Sinemet: A prescription drug used to treat Parkinson's Disease or sometimes Restless Leg Syndrome.

Soleus Muscle: A deep muscle in the calf that works with the Gastrocnemius Muscle to allow pushing downward with the toes.

Statins: A prescription drug used to lower Cholesterol to prevent cardiovascular disease. Unfortunately, it is a misconception that Cholesterol causes cardiovascular disease.

Subluxation: A Chiropractic concept describing the malposition of a joint, less than a dislocation, but enough to cause nerve irritation. The nerve irritation is caused by either nerve compression or proprioceptive disturbance.

Subliminal Infection (also called Subclinical Infection): An infection that is so minor that it does exhibit the typical signs of infection such as inflammation, pain and fever. However, it may produce other problems such as metabolic disturbances or disturbed reflexes.

Systemic Imbalance: A physiological or psychological stress that disturbs the metabolism such that it strains the homeostatic adaptive abilities of the body.

Telomere: The end section of the DNA strands that shorten each time a cell divides. When the Telomere becomes too short the cell involved will stop dividing.

Tennis Elbow: A painful condition of the lateral elbow often caused by repetitive motion of the arm such as in playing tennis or typing.

Thalamus: A part of the deep brain nuclei that serves as a relay and integration center for sensations from the body. Part of the Thalamus, the VPL, integrates pain and proprioception.

Therapy Localization: A Chiropractic technique discovered by Dr. George Goodheart. His discovery was that a strong muscle will weaken when a disturbed part of the body is touched, or a weak muscle will strengthen if the disturbed body area is related energetically to the weak muscle.

Tibialis Anterior: A muscle in the shins that dorsiflexes the foot.

Trematode: A microscopic worm that looks like a leaf, flat and pointed at both ends. They are also known as flukes or flat worms. They can cause many health problems including GI disturbances, lung problems, liver problems and possibly Cancer.

Vertebrae: A bone of the spinal column.

Virus: The smallest known life form.

Viscerosomatic reflexes: Reflexes between organs of the body and the muscular system. Typically a disturbed organ, such as the heart, will cause pain and muscle spasm.

Voll Testing: Dr. Reinhard Voll, MD in the 1940s developed a system of Electrodiagnostic Testing called EAV (Electrodiagnosis according to Voll) which is still in use today, especially in Europe. It has proved to be the for-runner of many number of evolving technologies such as the LSA.

VPL: An abbreviation for Ventralposteriolateral Nucleus of the Thalamus, a brain center that integrates feedback from the body for pain and proprioception.

Yohimbe: An herb that research has shown to be a true aphrodisiac.

Youth Span: As distinguished from lifespan, it represents the period in life until old age sets in.

Zippity Doo Dah: A whimsical tune from the Uncle Remus stories sung by such characters as Br'er Fox when life is doing especially well. Here it represents the sense of well being that manifests in peak health.

Index

About The Author

Dr. Robert Janda graduated from UC Berkley with a BA in Experimental Psychology in 1968. The year following graduation he stayed in the San Francisco area to study Gestalt Psychotherapy under the tutelage of Robert K. Hall, M.D. The following year he began studies in Clinical Psychology at California State University in Fresno. In 1972, he graduated with a Masters Degree in Clinical Psychology with a special interest in hypnosis and Jungian Psychology.

After an interlude, he moved to Los Angeles in 1976 to study acupuncture from Korean and Chinese practitioners and their American students. During this time he also took courses in Swedish Massage, Shiatsu, Acupressure and Jin Shin Do. He also studied Iridology and Nutrition with Bernard Jensen, DC, launching his lifelong interest in nutrition, which has continued to the present. In 1977, for one year, Dr. Janda worked as an acupuncturist at Harbor General Hospital Pain Clinic in San Pedro under Dr. Mok.

In 1978, Dr. Janda began studies in Chiropractic at the Los

Angeles College of Chiropractic. Starting the following year, and during his Chiropractic schooling, Dr. Janda began two years of seminars in Applied Kinesiology, which has become his special interest in the Chiropractic field. In 1980, also while still a student at the Chiropractic College, he began studies at the California College of Acupuncture in Los Angeles. Two years later he graduated from both institutions at the same time and received his Doctorate in Chiropractic.

Since that time he has been in private practice in Costa Mesa, California, practicing Chiropractic, Nutrition Therapy and Applied Kinesiology. For the past 17 years he has continued his education in Nutrition through numerous professional seminars. As a sidetrack, in 1988 he entered the Bruchion Art School in Los Angeles and studied Old Master Oil Painting for six years. He currently paints professionally on a part time basis.

In 1997, he began studies at the Rolf Institute in Boulder, Colorado and was certified in Rolfing Structural Integration the following year. This technique has been incorporated into his current practice. In 2002, Dr. Janda took the basic and advanced seminars in Dr. Nambudripad's Allergy Elimination Technique (NAET) and was certified in that technique. In 2003, Dr. Janda has continued his training through certification in the three areas of Active Release Technique (ART), the spine and upper and lower extremities. In November 2003, he participated as an ART doctor treating athletes in the Ironman contest in Kona, Hawaii.

Dr. Janda now practices in Costa Mesa and in Temecula, California. He has taken special interest in carpal tunnel and tendonitis symptomology and has developed effective procedures for diagnosing and resolving these problems. He also works on diverse musculoskelletal problems such as spinal injuries, whiplash, and athletic injuries. The Clinic acquired a DRX 9000 C for spinal decompression to rehabilitate spinal discs that are degenerate, bulging or ruptured. This technology will eliminate the need for most disc surgeries. Through the use of nutrition he treats metabolic and female health problems such as PMS, digestive problems and toxicity. He is also interested in strengthening immunity and promoting longevity as well as the prevention of serious health problems such as heart disease and cancer. Dr. Janda believes that psychological, nutritional and bio-mechanical factors are mutually interactive. His mode of practice is more akin to preventative Naturopathic Medicine although it includes conventional Chiropractic.

Robert L. Janda, MA, DC

Made in the USA
Charleston, SC
21 September 2011